Physiotherapeutic Management of Lumbar Spine Pathology

David MacDonald
Rick Jemmett

An evidence-based, best-practice clinical model incorporating prospective clinical reasoning, manual therapy and segmental stabilization exercises

novont health publishing limited · halifax · nova scotia · canada

Library and Archives Canada Cataloguing in Publication

MacDonald, David, 1972-
    Physiotherapeutic management of lumbar spine pathology : an evidence-based,
best-practice clinical model incorporating prospective clinical reasoning, manual therapy
and segmental stabilization exercises / David MacDonald, Rick Jemmett.

Includes bibliographical references and index.
ISBN 0-9688715-2-6

    1. Lumbar vertebrae--Diseases--Treatment. 2. Backache--Physical therapy.
I. Jemmett, Rick, 1961- II. Title.

RM701.M33 2005   617.5'64062
C2005-902609-X

Post Production	Rick Jemmett
Models	Brent Thompson, FCAMT; Joe Baldock, Cathy MacInnis, Sarah Murphy
Additional Illustrations	Margaret Galloway
Additional Photography	Wesley J Steeves

Printed in Canada

novont health publishing limited

Halifax, Canada B3H 4M8
902 423 4344

www.novonthealth.com
info@novonthealth.com

First Printing   April 2005

Knowledge in the various areas of scientific research and medical and rehabilitative professional practice is updated regularly. As new information becomes available, changes to clinical practice guidelines and the best-practice management of patients with pathology are inevitable. The authors and publisher have taken great care to ensure that the information presented is accurate, up-to-date and in keeping with the highest standards of practice at the time of publication. The author and publisher are not responsible for errors or omissions or for any consequences which may arise from application of the information in this book.

Physiotherapeutic Management of Lumbar Spine Pathology

An evidence-based, best-practice clinical model incorporating
prospective clinical reasoning, manual therapy and
segmental stabilization exercises

David MacDonald & Rick Jemmett

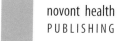

novont health
PUBLISHING

Dedicated to Mr. Robert MacDonald

... friend, colleague, gentleman, marathon runner, aspiring meteorologist and the owner and clinical director of Maritime Physiotherapy. We couldn't imagine a better place to practice the satisfying and humbling craft of orthopaedic physiotherapy. In your typically quiet fashion, you have set a unique standard in compassion and ethics; we are both honoured to have had the opportunity to work alongside you.

Our seemingly ever increasing time away from work to learn, dissect and teach and write is possible only through your unlimited patience and encouragement.

Thanks Rob.

contents

CHAPTER ONE
Towards A New Paradigm in Patient Management

CHAPTER TWO
Anatomy & Tri-Planar Segmental Biomechanics of the Lumbar Spine

CHAPTER THREE
Segmental Stability & Motor Control in the Lumbar Spine

CHAPTER FOUR
Clinical Reasoning & the Segmental Dysfunction Model

acknowledgements

A TEXTBOOK IS NEVER a solitary effort and this work is no exception. We are indebted to our undergraduate professors at the University of Toronto and Dalhousie University; they instilled in us a respect for those clinicians who pioneered orthopaedic manual therapy (and who did so without an extensive, clinically relevant literature base, the internet or Fed Ex) while at the same time encouraging us to embrace change and new ideas.

Over the years our many instructors, mentors and colleagues have made important contributions to the ideas which are now expressed in this text. It will be obvious to many that we have borrowed extensively from some very wise and observant manual therapy practitioners. We are either directly or indirectly indebted to Gregory Grieve, Cliff Fowler, David Lamb, Erl Pettman, Geoffrey Maitland, Duncan MacAuley, David Butler, Diane Lee, Jim Meadows and Wendy Aspinall.

An evidence-based clinical model would obviously not be possible without a large amount of multi-disciplinary research. The authors would like to acknowledge the important and often elegant work of Nik Bogduk, Jacek Cholewicki, JJ Crisco, Julie Hides, Paul Hodges, Gwen Jull, Lorimer Moseley, Thomas Oxland, Carolyn Richardson, Moshe Solomonow, and Andre Vleeming.

A specific note regarding the significant contributions to the field of spinal biomechanics by Dr. Manohar Panjabi is warranted. Panjabi's work over the past fifteen years has been fundamental to the development of a profound and novel understanding of spinal function and dysfunction. All who pursue this field of research will be influenced by the enlightened work of this fine scientist.

A special thank you to all the clinicians across Canada and in the United States and Australia who reviewed the final drafts and made helpful and always constructive criticisms of our work. Thank you as well to Anne Agur at the University of Toronto who was instrumental in our obtaining, dissecting and photographing the anatomic dissection material used in chapter two. Our sincere gratitude to Cathy MacInnis, Joe Baldock and Brent Thompson who modeled for the assessment and treatment chapters, enduring long photo shoots in a cold studio.

Finally, we wish to acknowledge the patience, encouragement and love of our significant others and families. Sharon, Eugene and Phyllis, who are missed, and Meagan, Jennifer, Wesley, Christa, Malcolm & Cory - without you this book would not have been possible nor nearly as worthwhile writing.

RJ & DM

preface

THE TOPIC OF THIS TEXT, not surprisingly, is the physiotherapeutic management of patients with lumbar pathology. However, as with any such clinical entity, the assessment and treatment of patients with symptoms secondary to lumbar spine dysfunction can hardly be considered a single 'topic'. Rather, the physiotherapeutic management of lumbar spine pathology requires our consideration of many collections of knowledge. Current research in anatomy, epidemiology, normal motor control, impaired motor control, biomechanics, clinical reasoning, pathology, psychology and clinical efficacy studies along with clinical experience must each be considered in the context of the pathological lumbar spine.

In the past fifteen years, a more predictable and clinically relevant model of the lumbar spine has emerged, largely through the efforts of researchers who began to ask the kinds of questions posed by clinicians over the past several decades. As clinicians on the sidelines watching this research unfold, it has been very interesting to watch the ball being advanced down field. If one goes back to the mid-1980s and begins with the work of Bergmark, Crisco, Gertzbein and Panjabi, one can easily trace the connections through the literature, observing how a single concept or finding developed in one lab was expanded upon or further refined in another. Twenty years later, a model of

the lumbar spine exists which can be regarded as 'evidence-based', and still hold up in the real world of the clinician.

This text is by no means a comprehensive dissertation on the topic of lumbar pathology. Readers will not find any discussion of pathologies such as osteoporosis, spinal infections, neoplasms, nor rheumatological diseases of the spine. We have purposefully avoided the topic of the dysfunctional pelvis as it has received expert attention in recent years. Our intention was to provide physiotherapy clinicians with a sound clinical model suitable for use with the patient who presents with symptoms suggestive of a deficit of the lumbar spine, its muscles and/or its motor control mechanisms. With this objective in mind, we feel we have provided a clinical model which will permit physiotherapists to manage their patients with lumbar pathology far more effectively than was the case with more traditional models.

In terms of the intended audience for the text, we feel that it should have broad application within the orthopaedic conservative-care community. We have not made any specific effort to write towards a certain 'target' reader. Instead, our intention was to describe a practical yet research-driven model of lumbar pathology management and let clinicians take from it what they will. Students in upper year orthopaedics courses will likely find it to be a thorough and demanding discussion. Clinicians with some exposure to *manual therapy* and *specific stabilization exercises* will hopefully find that the text helps them integrate their developing clinical knowledge and skill sets and appreciate more fully how it all 'fits together'. Clinicians who practice primarily from a functional conditioning perspective will find their paradigm challenged from both the theoretical and applied perspectives. Finally, expert clinicians will hopefully find aspects of this clinical model to be of interest as traditional concepts regarding spinal stability, clinical reasoning and the interpretation of certain *manual therapy* tests are considered against the backdrop of the current literature.

DM & RJ

introduction

Science is the tool of the Western mind and with it more doors can be opened than with bare hands. It is part and parcel of our knowledge and obscures our insight only when it holds that the understanding it provides is the only kind there is. C.G. Jung

JUNG'S COMMENTARY REGARDING the interactions between the scientific and the experiential seems especially insightful when considered within the context of a discussion of lumbar spine pathology and its management by manual therapy clinicians. It makes the argument that ultimately, science provides more complete and effective solutions, while suggesting that the challenges inherent in clinical practice often define the nature and scope of the most compelling problems. It speaks of the need for clinicians and researchers to acknowledge the value and importance of each discipline and calls for a balanced approach to clinical decision making. This commentary also serves as an ideal summary for the key objectives of this text: that is, to develop and present a clinical model of lumbar spine pathology which is both evidence-based and clinically relevant.

Only twenty years ago, any suggestion that a clinical model of the lumbar spine could be both evidence-based and clinically relevant probably seemed unlikely to many manual therapy clinicians. Fortunately, a dramatic turn in the course of the literature occurred in the late 1980's and early 1990's resulting in a set of circumstances which now provide for such a model. Indeed, our discussion of lumbar spine pathology and its management takes place at a time when evolving research adds to our understanding of the etiology and behaviour of this condition on at least a bi-weekly basis.

This text will present a clinical model of lumbar spine pathology and management which may well be seen by many clinicians as unique, and perhaps even radical. This clinical model will challenge conventional beliefs regarding both the nature of lumbar dysfunction and the management of patients with lower quadrant symptoms. Although the model requires a re-evaluation of many long-accepted concepts, it nonetheless supports certain fundamental clinical tenets. Furthermore, the model is far more predictive of the clinical patterns with which our patients present than are more traditional models. While novel, its foundations are sound. It has evolved secondary to substantive changes in both clinical practice and the scientific literature.

From the scientific perspective, a wealth of multi-disciplinary and clinically relevant evidence has developed over the past fifteen years. Careful consideration of this research affords the clinician a more comprehensive understanding of lumbar pathology and its symptomatic manifestation in various patient presentations or clinical patterns. Clinically, physical therapists have become, in many jurisdictions, primary care providers of neuro-musculoskeletal care to the general public. As such, physical therapists have become *diagnostic clinicians* rather than the therapeutic technicians of forty years ago. This evolution necessitates the application of higher level clinical reasoning models. Fortunately, such management models exist and are easily adapted to physical therapy practice. Before looking more closely at the current situation, it is useful to briefly consider the evolution of the physical therapy profession over the past several decades.

For example, orthopaedic physical therapists played a very limited diagnostic role in the management of their patients. Orthopaedic pathology was managed by physicians using a classical pathoanatomical model, a model which assumed that some identifiable structure could be determined to be the source of the patient's pain. In terms of spinal pathology, the pathoanatomical model gave rise to diagnoses such as facet joint syndrome, discogenic back pain, lumbar strain and degenerative disc disease. Treatment, whether surgical or conservative, was designed to lessen the stresses placed on the suspected pathological structure. It was expected that the structure would eventually heal and that the patient's symptoms would resolve. At that time, the majority of a physical therapist's caseload consisted of patients with either post-surgical or post-traumatic pathology. The need for physical therapists to possess any significant diagnostic ability was minimal. The patient's physician or surgeon would develop the diagnosis (and often the treatment plan) while the physical therapist would develop a 'problem list' during their initial visit with the patient.

For example, a post-surgical patient having recently undergone a discectomy might then see the physical therapist, who would likely note a variety of problems such as pain, decreased range of motion, and an inability to perform normal daily activities. The physical therapist would then set out to correct these 'discrete' problems one by one, treating their pain, improving their range of mo-

tion and finding ways to help them return to more normal levels of function. In post-surgical and post-traumatic populations, this approach continues to work well.

In 2005, the typical working environment for physical therapists has changed in two significant ways. First, many orthopaedic physical therapists now see a greater proportion of patients with non-traumatic, non-surgical conditions. Second, an increasing number of jurisdictions have granted direct access privileges to physical therapists, giving them far more responsibility for determining the patient's diagnosis. The significance of these changes is dramatic. The profession has moved from a working situation in which the diagnosis was relatively obvious and provided by another clinician, to one in which the physical therapist is responsible for determining the diagnosis in a population of patients whose underlying pathology might not be quite as straight forward as had been predicted by the pathoanatomical model.

In the past decade, a large body of research regarding the etiology, epidemiology and management of lumbar pathology has been published. Older concepts of spinal function and stability have been revised as more recent research has demonstrated that the spinal column is inherently unstable (Crisco, 1989; Oxland & Panjabi, 1992) and therefore in need of ongoing coordinated support from the muscular and nervous systems (Panjabi, 1992a; Cholewicki et al, 1997; Hodges & Moseley, 2003). There is much evidence that the spinal column, spinal muscles and nervous system function in such an integrated manner that pathology or dysfunction in one system will likely lead to some degree of pathology or dysfunction in the remaining two (Hodges & Richardson, 1996; McGill, 1997; Solomonow et al, 1999; Panjabi, 2003). Despite the fact that injured tissues do heal, there is evidence to suggest that some degree of muscular deficit persists following spinal surgery (Rantanen, 1993) and beyond the resolution of symptoms in acute onset low back pain (Hides et al, 1996). This consistent pattern of multi-system dysfunction contradicts the traditional pathoanatomical model in which a single structure was assumed to have been responsible for the patient's symptoms.

Over a similar period, epidemiological and clinical outcomes studies have reported that the conservative management of acute, chronic or recurrent low back pain is frequently unpredictable and often ineffective (Von Korff & Saunders, 1996; van den Hoogen et al, 1997; Croft et al, 1998; Mannion et al, 1999; Bogduk, 2004; Frost et al, 2004; Hurley et al, 2004). While there may be reasonable concerns regarding the extent to which some of these studies satisfied the strictest criteria for sound research, they do in fact report on the efficacy of conservative care as it is practised in the real-world. Outcomes studies of more evidence-based clinical models - models similar to that described in this text - have demonstrated that such approaches may be significantly more effective at improving pain and function in chronic low back pain (O'Sullivan et al, 1997; Moseley et al, 2002) and reducing a person's risk of future episodes of low back pain (Hides et al, 2001).

In our opinion, these fundamental changes regarding the literature and the realities of clinical practice necessitate a re-evaluation of our approach to the management of patients with lumbar pathology. The clinician who must independently manage patients with lumbar spine pathology requires a comprehensive appreciation for the multi-system dysfunction which develops in the majority of patients. Furthermore, clinicians require a diagnostic approach grounded in prospective clinical reasoning to be capable of developing an accurate appreciation for the dysfunction present in individual patients. As will be discussed in later sections of this text, lumbar dysfunction does not confine itself symptomatically to the lumbar region. With an appreciation for spinal biomechanics and neurophysiological issues, and an ability to apply sound manual therapy principles, the clinician's ability to manage patients with a variety of lower quadrant complaints will be markedly improved.

The objective of this text is to describe an evidence-based clinical model regarding the management of patients with lumbar spine pathology. This model, the *Segmental Dysfunction Model*, integrates the most recent biomechanical, neurophysiological, anatomical and epidemiological evidence with current concepts regarding manual therapy and clinical reasoning. With appropriate application of the model, the authors anticipate that clinicians will realize more predictable, consistent and effective clinical outcomes.

This text is divided into eight chapters. The first chapter compares the pathoanatomical, bio-psychosocial and segmental dysfunction models in terms of predictive validity and the extent to which each is compatible with the current literature. The second and third chapters detail the basic sciences research fundamental to the segmental dysfunction model. This includes an overview of the clinically relevant anatomy and segmental spinal bio-mechanics, a review of Panjabi's hypotheses and experimental findings regarding stability, clinical segmental instability and the relationships between spinal pathology and the so-called *neutral zone*. Chapter three also includes a discussion of motor control issues as related to both the normal and the dysfunctional lumbar spine.

The fourth chapter reviews the topic of clinical reasoning, specifically the retrospective and prospective models of clinical reasoning, in the context of current orthopaedic physiotherapy practice. The second half of this chapter describes in detail the segmental dysfunction model, which is based upon the material presented in chapters two and three. Chapter five details a comprehensive manual therapy model of lumbar spine assessment. This includes both the subjective and physical examinations and a discussion of the rationale underlying each manual therapy test. The technical considerations for each of the tests are presented using written descriptions and photographs. The sixth chapter is devoted to the treatment of the patient with lumbar dysfunction. Practical descriptions and photographs of the articular, motor control and neurodynamic interventions are presented to facilitate their clinical application. Chapter seven presents a variety of lumbar case studies. The objective of this chapter is to present the segmental dysfunction model in practice, demonstrating its application with actual patients as treated by the authors. The final chapter presents a series of invited commentaries. Although common in the peer-reviewed literature, we are not aware of the inclusion of such a section in a textbook, certainly not in the physiotherapy domain. Our intention with this final chapter is to help foster a necessary transparency within the physiotherapy literature. If we are to make the claim that this text represents an 'evidence-based, best-practice' clinical model, then we should be prepared to subject our work to a variety of expert and considered opinions. It is our hope that this chapter will stimulate debate and draw out a range of perspectives on the always contentious topic of lumbar pathology.

CHAPTER **ONE**

towards a new paradigm in patient management

The Pathoanatomical, Biopsychosocial and Segmental Dysfunction Models of Low Back Pain

MODELS ARE USED EXTENSIVELY in science, business, medicine and many other areas of human activity. A model may be defined as a thoughtful, evidence-based analysis of a set of data, often expressed in words, as a series of mathematical equations or as software code. Regardless of the activity, models attempt to explain or predict how something will occur or evolve in the real world. For example, a business model is an analysis of all the known factors which might affect the viability of a new business venture. Einstein's *Theory of Relativity* is a model of how the universe functions. Models, especially those in the natural sciences, are also quite fluid; they are expected to evolve as new data becomes available.

In all circumstances, the utility of a model is determined by the accuracy with which that model predicts events in the real world. Not surprisingly, the ability of a model to accurately predict real world behaviour is largely dependent upon the quality and comprehensiveness of the data used to construct the model. Consider a business model which failed to account for 40% of the long-term costs associated with the delivery of a new product line. It is likely that the model would ultimately prove to have been a poor predictor of the product's viability and would, in retrospect, be considered a poor model. Hundreds of years ago, the clinical model for 'sudden, severe lower right abdominal pain' had more to do with an imbalance of humours than with an inflamed appendix. The current clinical model for 'sudden, severe lower right abdominal pain' has proven to be vastly more predictive and thus more clinically useful.

In orthopaedics, models are used to help clinicians conceptualize, explain and manage the types of problems and symptoms encountered in clinical practice. Two types of orthopaedic models - biomechanical and clinical - are familiar to most clinicians. Biomechanical models, with their basis in physics and engineering, attempt to predict, *via* mathematical equations, the normal and/or abnormal behaviour of some biomechanical system such as the foot, the shoulder complex or the lumbar spine. Clinical models integrate multi-disciplinary scientific research with clinical findings and experience. The objective of any clinical model is improved patient management. The three clinical models we will consider in this chapter are the pathoanatomical, the biopsychosocial and the segmental dysfunction models.

The Pathoanatomical Model

DURING THE PAST SEVERAL decades the conservative (i.e., non-surgical) management of lumbar spine pathology has been based on the *pathoanatomical* model, a clinical approach in which some identifiable anatomical structure was considered to be the primary source of the patient's symptoms. The pathological structure might be articular, muscular, neural, vascular or visceral. Within this model, diagnoses such as discogenic back pain, zygapophysial joint sprain, and lumbar muscle strain are common. The physiotherapeutic management of patients with lumbar spine pathology has typically been structured to minimize or alleviate the mechanical or chemical stresses affecting the structure identified as being pathologic.

For example, if the patient were diagnosed with discogenic low back pain, treatment would often involve an anti-flexion protocol, mechanical traction and repeated lumbar extension. The patient would later be progressed through a program of general conditioning exercises, as tolerated. However, if the diagnosis of zyga-pophysial joint sprain was developed for a patient, they would likely be treated using an anti-extension protocol. Again, the patient would eventually be provided with a general conditioning program. If the clinician arrived at a diagnosis of muscle strain, the patient might be given some combination of therapeutic flexion and extension activities and then progressed along a course of general conditioning exercises.

Despite the apparent logic inherent in the pathoanatomical approach, and the fact that in some circumstances it performs reasonably well (for instance, in post-surgical populations), significant limitations regarding the predictive accuracy of the pathoanatomical model have been identified. One of these, a diagnostic issue, concerns the physical examination's inability to consistently and properly identify either the structure or the lesion-type (Mooney, 1989). MacNab has shown that patients with very similar forms of spinal pathology present with a wide variety of signs and symptoms and that the same set of signs and symptoms may arise from a number of different pathologic structures (MacNab, 1971). Likewise, spondylolisthesis and 'non-specific' low back pain have been reported as being highly similar in terms of their clinical findings (Moller et al, 2000). Clinicians - both physiotherapists and physicians - are well aware of the frequency with which their physical examination findings fail to correlate with findings on MRI, CT or arthroscopy in both spinal and peripheral populations. In one recent study comparing physical and arthroscopic examination, clinical tests were only moderately predictive of the findings at surgery (Holtby & Razmjou, 2004). It would appear then that the pathoanatomically-based clinical examination is not capable of predicting the specific structural origin of a patient's symptoms as accurately and consistently as clinicians might expect (Varamini & Jam 2005a).

A second and related limitation involves the pathoanatomical model's capacity for prognosis. Spitzer and colleagues reported that "prognosis has become a matter of opinion and not of fact" (Spitzer et al, 1987). Regardless of the difficulties in doing so, it is important for clinicians to develop an accurate prognosis for their patients with low back pain. A sound prognosis facilitates a more effective and efficient management plan and generates realistic therapeutic objectives. However, the development of an accurate prognosis is closely linked to the existence of an accurate diagnosis. If the clinician's ability to accurately identify both the pathologic structure and the degree to which it is injured is poor, any attempt to predict a patient's outcome based upon this 'diagnosis' will be similarly limited. Indeed, in regard to non-specific low back pain, a number of epidemiological and therapeutic outcomes studies support this contention (van den Hoogen et al, 1997; Frost et al, 2004).

On an individual basis it can be difficult for the clinician to predict which patient will recover in a timely fashion, which patient will develop an episodic pattern of low back pain and which patient will go on to experience truly chronic symptoms (Von Korff & Saunders, 1996; van den Hoogen et al, 1997; Croft et al, 1998). While epidemiologists may be content to describe how non-specific low back pain behaves across populations, clinicians need to understand how individual patients will progress in terms of timelines and extent of recovery. Unfortunately, the pathoanatomical model, with its fundamental deficits in terms of diagnostic precision, does not allow the clinician to develop a dependable prognosis in the majority of cases.

Given the problems associated with forming a sound diagnosis and prognosis, the patho-anatomical management of patients with low back pain is often guided more by the patient's symptomatic presentation than by any form of predictive and clinically-reasoned measure. This can result in the clinician employing a variety of treatment 'options' until the patient's symptoms subside. Typically, whichever intervention coincides with the patient's symptomatic improvement is assumed to have been responsible for this resolution. However, the same intervention employed with another patient, even one with a similar pathoanatomical presentation, may be unlikely to lead to a similar outcome. In our experience, both as clinicians and as educators, this unpredictability is a source of significant frustration for both the patient and the clinician.

In addition to concerns regarding the pathoanatomical model's lack of predictive capacity, recent research suggests that a 'single structure' concept of orthopaedic pathology is not tenable. As originally hypothesized by Panjabi (Panjabi, 1992) orthopaedic lumbar pathology necessarily entails a simultaneous and inter-related dysfunction of the articular, muscular and neural systems. Subsequent research has lent support to this multi-system model of lumbar spine pathology (Rantanen et al, 1993; Hides et al, 1994; Hides et al, 1996; Hodges & Richardson, 1996; Zhao et al, 2000; Yoshihara et al, 2001; McGill et al, 2003). The current evidence points to a model which requires the neural, muscular and articular systems to function in concert, and in a highly integrated fashion. This integration is such that pathology in one system invariably leads to dysfunction and compensatory adaptation in other systems. Thus, while a single anatomical structure may well become pathologic (e.g., an intervertebral disc herniation or a zygapophysial joint capsule injury) this pathology will lead to dysfunction in other related systems. Interestingly, this recent research regarding spinal pathology dovetails nicely with older research regarding peripheral joints such as the knee (de Andrade, 1965; Spencer, 1984).

Summary

Based on the criteria for a sound model as outlined above, the pathoanatomical model of lumbar spine pathology often fails to be predictive in terms of diagnosis, prognosis and efficient management. Its efficacy is further undermined by its inability to account for the most recent research supporting a multi-system model of neuromusculoskeletal pathology. In light of these shortcomings, it is difficult to support the pathoanatomical model as a basis for the physiotherapeutic management of patients with lumbar spine pathology. Hopefully this will be of some comfort to those many clinicians who remain frustrated, despite their best efforts, with the assessment and treatment of patients with low back pain; the problem may well reside more with the model than with its application.

The Biopsychosocial Model

To some extent, the problems associated with the pathoanatomical model in the setting of lumbar spine pathology prompted the development of the biopsychosocial model of low back pain. Certainly, the high costs associated with managing a small subset of patients who experience significant functional disability secondary to ongoing low back pain (Spengler et al, 1986; Schultz et al, 2002) have spawned a large body of literature focused on the psychological and behavioural aspects of chronic low back pain. Since the mid-1980's, a growing series of studies have reported on the relationships between psychosocial factors, chronic low back pain and disability (Spengler et al, 1986; Krause et al, 1998; Schultz et al, 2002). Systematic reviews of this large body of research have also been published (Hoogendoorn et al, 2000; Pincus et al, 2002a).

The current literature regarding the bio-psychosocial model is concerned primarily with those patients who develop significant disability secondary to some undetectable physical impairment (Pincus et al, 2002a). A number of studies have found that such patients are in the minority, despite the fact that their cases account for the majority of the costs associated with the management of chronic low back pain (Spengler et al, 1986; Murphy & Courtney, 2000). A primary objective of this research has been the identification of those psychosocial factors which may be screened for clinically and which best predict disability secondary to low back pain (Fransen et al, 2002). Unfortunately, in this regard, there is still much disagreement in the literature. Schultz and colleagues reported that cognitive items such as the patient's expectations of recovery and perceptions of current health status were most strongly predictive of future disability (Schultz et al, 2002). Conversely, psychological factors such as depression and anxiety have also been reported to be strongly associated with chronic low back pain related disability (Pincus et al, 2002a). Another psychosocial factor, fear of movement-related pain, has also been described as being highly predictive of disability (Pincus et al, 2002a).

The following quote describes the primary assumptions which form the foundation of the biopsychosocial model (Pincus et al, 2002b):

"1. Impairment, pain and disability are conceptually related, but are also distinct.

2. Impairments (such as disc prolapse) are not caused by psychosocial factors, whereas the perception of pain is always subjective and is influenced readily by such factors.

3. The reporting of injuries and pain, and the seeking of health care, usually is mediated by the complex interaction of medical, work-related beliefs and behaviour and other psychosocial factors.

4. Disability, including work loss and reduction in activity, is commonly influenced by a diverse range of psychosocial factors. These factors include attitudes and beliefs held by the patient, behaviour, compensation and litigation issues, diagnosis and the behaviour of treatment providers, emotions, such as fear or low mood, family member's behaviour, such as a solicitous spouse, and work factors.

5. The presence of specific disease does not mean that psychosocial factors are unimportant."

The biopsychosocial model of low back pain is an evolving attempt to understand the interactions between the psychological and behavioural factors influencing the course of recovery in all instances of low back pain. In the broadest sense, every person who experiences low back pain (or any form of physical pathology) filters that experience through their own unique 'biopsychosocial lens' (Drinkwater, 2003). Whereas one individual's 'lens' may permit them to conceptualize their pain as an annoyance as they continue to lead a more or less normal and functional life, another person's 'lens' may facilitate a cycle of fear, catastrophizing and a continued state of hypervigilance which greatly interferes with their ability to participate fully in normal daily activities. At the opposite end of this spectrum are those patients who minimize the severity of their pathology, sometimes to the point where they put themselves at risk for more significant problems.

As noted above, although a variety of psychosocial factors have been identified as being related to outcomes, it is still not known which of these is most strongly correlated with the development of chronic disability. Thus, from the perspective of the model's predictive ability, the psychosocial variables which should be screened for have yet to be conclusively identified. In terms of its basic foundations, few clinicians would dispute the fundamental idea that psychosocial factors affect recovery, both positively and negatively. However, we must recognize that the biopsychosocial model is an incomplete model as it considers only the psychosocial aspects of disability. In recent years, convincing evidence demonstrating the presence of 'organic' pathology in patients with chronic low back pain has been reported. Briefly, this pathology includes a wide range of muscular changes involving the control of certain muscles of the spinal column (Hodges, 2003), persistent histochemical changes (Rantanen et al, 1993) and reductions in cross sectional area (Danneels et al, 2000) as well as changes in the central and peripheral nervous systems (Devor & Seltzer, 1999; Doubell et al, 1999). All or any of these may predispose patients to ongoing pain.

Summary

The biopsychosocial model considers the impact of a variety of psychosocial factors on the course of low back pain related disability. While a number of important factors have been identified, it is not yet known which of these is most strongly correlated with the development of such disability. Despite this lack of consensus, the potential significance of these factors requires physiotherapy clinicians to develop at least an appreciation for each patient's psychosocial status.

The biopsychosocial model has much to offer regarding the management of patients with significant disability secondary to chronic back pain. Nonetheless it is a somewhat incomplete model. It is concerned only with psychosocial variables and only with a relatively small subset of the low back pain population. Clinicians will recall that the majority of patients with back pain do not have *chronic* pain nor do they become markedly disabled by their symptoms. Furthermore, there is now good evidence demonstrating a series of persistent 'organic' deficits in people with recurrent and chronic back pain (please see chapter 3). Thus, the biopsychosocial model should not be considered as a viable approach to the management of patients with recurrent or episodic low back pain who often remain quite functional in terms of their ADLs, occupational responsibilities and sports activities.

The Segmental Dysfunction Model

GIVEN THE PROBLEMS associated with the pathoanatomical model and the limitations of the biopsychosocial model, it is apparent that clinicians require a more predictive, evidence-based and comprehensive model with which to approach the management of patients with low back pain. Over the past fifteen years, a significant amount of research has been published which can be drawn upon to develop such a model. Recent anatomical, biomechanical and neurophysiological research, along with higher level clinical reasoning concepts, provide for a model which is both evidence-based and clinically sound. This research is discussed in detail in later sections of this text. At this point, it is sufficient to simply list several of the key premises upon which the segmental dysfunction model (SDM) is based and provide an outline of the model. The SDM is described in detail in chapter four following a discussion of clinical reasoning theory.

Foundations of the SDM:

1. The belief that a clinical examination can consistently and accurately identify the primary anatomical structure or tissue responsible for the patient's symptoms is no longer supportable.

2. The majority of lumbar spine pathology involves a predictable set of interdependent deficits affecting the osseoligamentous and neuromuscular systems. This pattern of deficits develops regardless of whether the underlying pathology involves the intervertebral disc, the zygapophysial joint tissues, a spinal ligament, a spinal muscle or the vertebra itself.

3. The deficit affecting the osseoligamentous system results in an alteration of the normal intersegmental stiffness characteristics of the pathological segment.

4. The neuromuscular changes evident in the presence of lumbar spine pathology include impaired control of the deep segmental muscles coupled with an excessive, compensatory activation of the multi-segmental muscles of the lumbar region. There is evidence that these deficits may persist indefinitely, and regardless of whether the patient's symptoms resolve, continue or recur intermittently.

5. The articular and neuromuscular deficits which develop secondary to lumbar spine pathology may result in a wide range of patient presentations, with symptoms experienced in the lumbar region, the lower extremity or both.

6. The traditional skill set and scope of practice of orthopaedic physical therapists includes the clinical assessment of articular stiffness and neuromuscular function.

7. The traditional skill set and scope of practice of orthopaedic physical therapists includes the treatment of articular and neuromuscular dysfunction.

8. The incorporation of *prospective clinical reasoning* within the context of the segmental dysfunction model will facilitate more predictable and efficacious management of patients with lumbar spine pathology.

Overview of the Segmental Dysfunction Model

The SDM has been developed specifically to address the shortcomings inherent in the pathoanatomical and biopsychosocial models. Its main objective is to facilitate the clinician's ability to effectively and efficiently manage the patient with lumbar spine pathology. The model has a greater correspondence with the existing literature and an improved ability to predict and account for the various patient presentations encountered in clinical practice. Indeed, the SDM allows for an evidence-based classification system in low back pain, secondary to the identification of the primary underlying dysfunction present in the majority of patients with lumbar pathology.

As will be detailed in chapter three, there is currently excellent evidence that both non-specific and discogenic lumbar spine pathology consistently involves two fundamental deficits which occur together and which result in a wide range of symptomatic presentations. These deficits are a change in the normal stiffness characteristics of the lumbar spine and a loss of normal motor control affecting the muscles of the lumbar region. More specifically, this change in spinal stiffness typically involves a reduction in segmental stiffness at the symptom generating segment. The alterations in motor control are characterized by impaired activation of the deep segmental muscles along with a compensatory increase in activation of the multi-segmental lumbar muscles. These osseo-ligamentous and neuromuscular deficits are proposed to be key pathomechanical features underlying most instances of non-specific and discogenic low back pain.

The SDM draws extensively upon existing 'manual therapy' theory and skills. However, the SDM does necessitate a re-evaluation of many traditional manual therapy tests and treatment techniques in terms of interpretation and utilization. This will be discussed in detail throughout chapters four, five and six.

The Segmental Dysfunction Model allows the clinician to:

1. Identify the primary symptom generating segment.

2. Develop a clinical appreciation for the extent and pattern of articular dysfunction affecting the primary symptom generating segment.

3. Develop a clinical appreciation for the extent and pattern of neuromuscular dysfunction occurring in the vicinity of the primary symptom generating segment.

4. Develop a clinical appreciation for the extent and pattern of articular dysfunction occurring at segments adjacent to the primary symptom generating segment.

5. Utilize prospective clinical reasoning in the development of a clinical diagnosis, prognosis and management plan.

Summary

The segmental dysfunction model is a clinical model of lumbar spine pathology and its management. It is an integrated model blending existing research along with clinical findings and physiotherapeutic expertise. As with most clinical models, 'clinical experience' is used to fill in the gaps in the existing literature. However, the past fifteen years have seen remarkable progress in terms of clinically relevant research - research which predicts and accounts for the clinical patterns observed both in individual patients and within patient populations. There are now far fewer gaps to be filled. This new research allows clinicians to re-evaluate some of our traditional beliefs about the lumbar spine and the management of patients with lumbar pathology. We are confident that clinicians who can apply the model in their clinical practice will realize greatly improved outcomes in terms of predictability and overall success.

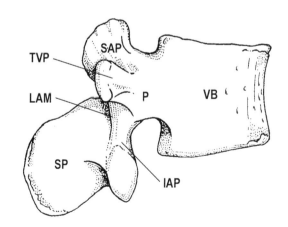

CHAPTER TWO

anatomy & tri-planar segmental biomechanics

Prior to conducting any form of assessment or treatment of the lumbar spine, it is of the utmost importance that the clinician possess a thorough understanding of the anatomy and segmental biomechanics of the region. A comprehensive understanding of the relevant lumbar anatomy and segmental biomechanics is prerequisite to an understanding of the normal and pathological behaviour of the spine, and the successful management of patients with lumbar dysfunction. As an exhaustive review is beyond the scope of this book, the reader is referred to the excellent text by Bogduk, *Clinical Anatomy of the Lumbar Spine and Sacrum, 3rd Ed.*

Clinically Relevant Anatomy of the Lumbar Spine

Anatomy of an Individual Lumbar Vertebra

THE FIVE LUMBAR vertebrae are relatively consistent in size and shape. Considered from a lateral view the primary features of an individual lumbar vertebra, from anterior to posterior, are as follows: the body, the pedicle, and the posterior elements,

consisting of the transverse process, the superior articular process, the inferior articular process, the lamina and the spinous process (figure 2.1).

The pedicles attach the vertebral body to the posterior elements. As the vertebral body is the primary weightbearing component of a lumbar vertebra and the posterior elements act largely as attachment points for muscles and fascial structures, the pedicles function to transmit forces between

Figure 2.1 Typical lumbar vertebra, lateral view from the right. VB = vertebral body; P = pedicle; SAP = superior articular process; TVP = transverse process; IAP = inferior articular process; LAM = lamina; SP = spinous process (*adapted from Bogduk, Clinical Anatomy of the Lumbar Spine and Sacrum, 3rd Ed., 1997 with permission*).

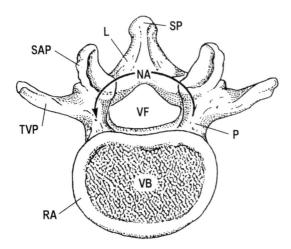

Figure 2.2 Typical lumbar vertebra, superior view. SP = spinous process; L = lamina; SAP = superior articular process; TVP = transverse process; RA = ring apophysis; P = pedicle; NA = neural arch; VF = vertebral foramen; VB = vertebral body (*adapted from Bogduk, Clinical Anatomy of the Lumbar Spine and Sacrum, 3rd Ed., 1997 with permission*).

the vertebral body and the posterior elements. The lamina may be considered as a 'bridge' or a 'weight-bearing wall' between the superior and inferior articular processes in a cranial to caudal direction, and between the spinous and transverse processes in a posterior to anterior direction.

In addition, the neural arch and the vertebral foramen are also appreciated *via* a superior view (figure 2.2). The neural arch is composed of the pedicles and laminae on both the right and left sides of the vertebra. The neural arch, along with the posterior aspect of the vertebral body, surrounds the vertebral foramen, protecting the delicate neural tissues within.

Anatomy of an Individual Lumbar Motion Segment

The terms 'motion segment', 'mobile segment', and 'functional spinal unit' are used by different authors to describe the composite structure of two adjacent vertebrae, their shared inter-vertebral disc and the ligaments which act on these structures (figure 2.3). The term *motion segment* is used throughout this text.

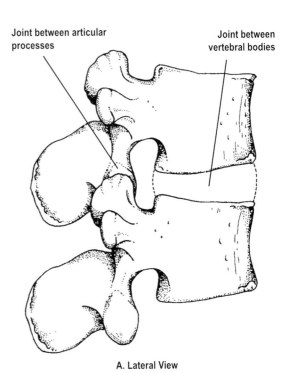

Joint between articular processes

Joint between vertebral bodies

A. Lateral View

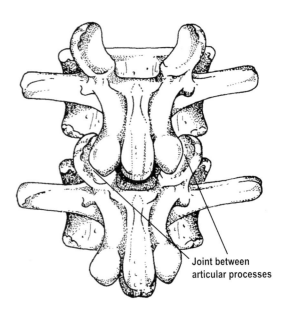

Joint between articular processes

B. Posterior View

Figure 2.3 Lateral and posterior views of a typical lumbar motion segment demonstrating the interbody and zygapophysial joints (*from Bogduk, Clinical Anatomy of the Lumbar Spine and Sacrum, 3rd Ed, 1997 with permission*).

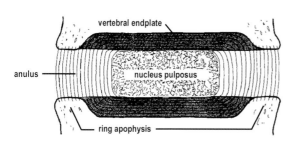

Figure 2.4 Detailed structure of the intervertebral disc (*from Bogduk, Clinical Anatomy of the Lumbar Spine and Sacrum, 3rd Ed, 1997 with permission*).

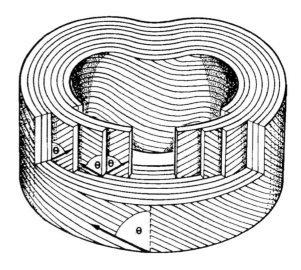

Figure 2.5 The structure of the anulus fibrosus (*from Bogduk, Clinical Anatomy of the Lumbar Spine and Sacrum, 3rd Ed, 1997 with permission*).

A lumbar motion segment has three distinct articulations: the interbody joint and the two zygapophysial joints. The interbody joint consists of the articulation of the superior and inferior vertebral bodies *via* the vertebral endplates and the intervening intervertebral disc. The zygapophysial joints (z-joints) are formed by the articulations between the superior and inferior articular processes and the capsule which surrounds them.

The Intervertebral Disc

The intervertebral disc consists of the centrally located nucleus pulposus which is surrounded by the anulus fibrosus. Both are encased by the superior and inferior vertebral endplates, also considered to be components of the intervertebral disc (figure 2.4) (Bogduk, 1997a). The nucleus pulposus is a semi-fluid, composed of cartilage cells, collagen and ground substance. Its composition allows the nucleus pulposus to deform under load, yet maintain its volume. Under load it will deform and disperse this load in all directions. Spinal loads are dispersed into the vertebral endplates superiorly and inferiorly, and into the anulus fibrosis laterally.

The anulus fibrosus is composed of collagen fibres, organized in ten to twenty concentrically organized sheets or *lamellae* (figure 2.5). The lamellae are consistently oriented at 65 degrees to the vertical yet their direction of orientation alternates in each successive lamellae. In terms of its internal to external dimensions, the anulus is thicker at the anterolateral aspect of the disc and thinner posteriorly. The anulus, having a greater diameter than the vertebral endplate, attaches to the superior and inferior vertebrae of the motion segment *via* the vertebral endplate and the ring apophysis, the outermost rim of the superior and inferior surfaces of the vertebral body. The vertebral endplates are composed of both hyaline cartilage and fibrocartilage. They are strongly attached to the anulus but less so to the vertebral body. As such, they can be torn away from the vertebral body with sufficient trauma (MacNab, 1977).

Mechanical and Neurological Functions of the Intervertebral Disc

The primary mechanical functions of the disc are the dispersion of compressive loads and the control of shear forces in three planes of motion. The hydraulic properties of the nucleus permit the disc to disperse the loads associated with weight-bearing and muscle contraction across a larger surface area. With the normal age-related degenerative changes which affect the nucleus, the ability of the intervertebral disc to perform this important function is impaired. While relatively recent studies have shown the lumbar disc and ligaments to be tolerant of loads far below those associated with physiological movement (Panjabi et al, 1998), the disc nonetheless provides a necessary degree of segmental motion control.

In addition, the intervertebral disc functions as part of the neurological system. Mechanoreceptors are found throughout the intervertebral disc, thus the disc is expected to provide proprioceptive feedback to the central nervous system regarding the dynamic mechanical status of the disc. While little is presently known regarding the precise nature of this proprioceptive input, emerging research has begun to illustrate the importance of this type of feedback in the activation of the paraspinal musculature (Indahl et al, 1997; Solomonow, 1998).

The Lumbar Zygapophysial Joints

The zygapophysial joints (z-joints) of the lumbar spine are formed of the superior and inferior articular processes and a fibrous joint capsule. As with typical synovial joints, a layer of synovium lines the internal surface of the joint capsule. A volume of intra-articular fat and as many as three types of meniscal structures are found within each z-joint.

The orientation of the z-joints significantly affects the biomechanics of the motion segment. Anatomical studies have indentified some variation in the shape and orientation of the lumbar z-joints between segmental levels and between individuals. The shape of the articular surfaces have been described as either flat, 'C'-shaped, or 'J'-shaped (figure 2.6). Regardless of their shape, the orientation of the articular surfaces tends to be more sagittal in the upper lumbar spine and becomes essentially coronal at L5-S1. The more sagittal the orientation, the less the segment is able to rotate, while a more coronal orientation is better suited to rotation. The coronal orientation of the L5-S1 z-joints, along with the attachment of the iliolumbar ligament at the L5 vertebra, allows the segment some degree of controlled rotation, with limited anterior translation in the sagittal plane. This restriction of anterior translation is essential

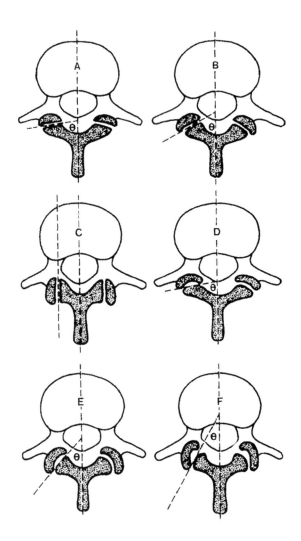

Figure 2.6 The variation in shape and orientation of the lumbar zygapophysial joints. A = flat joints oriented nearly perpendicular to the sagittal plane. B = curved joints oriented at approximately 60 degrees to the sagittal plane. C = flat joints oriented along the sagittal plane. D = curved joints oriented nearly perpendicular to the sagittal plane. E = a 'c'-shaped joint. F = a 'j'-shaped joint (*from Bogduk, Clinical Anatomy of the Lumbar Spine and Sacrum, 3rd Ed, 1997 with permission*).

given the steep angle (approximately 45 degrees) between the fifth lumbar and first sacral vertebrae.

Ligaments of the Lumbar Motion Segment

The primary ligaments of the lumbar motion segment are the anterior longitudinal, the posterior longitudinal, the ligamentum flavum, and the in-

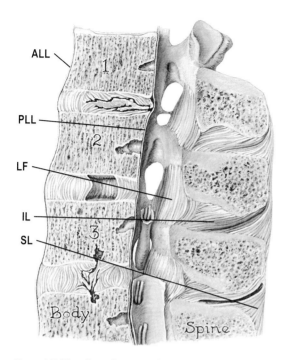

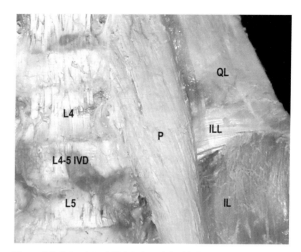

Figure 2.9 Anterolateral (right) view of the L4-5 motion segment. L4 = position of the body of the L4 vertebra. L4-5 IVD = L4-5 intervertebral dsc. L5 = position of the body of the L5 vertebra. QL = quadratus lumborum. P = psoas. IL = iliacus. ILL = iliolumbar ligament, superior and anterior components.

Figure 2.7 The primary ligaments of the lumbar spine. ALL = anterior longitudinal ligament; PLL = posterior longitudinal ligament; LF = ligamentum flavum; IL = interspinous ligament; SL = supraspinous ligament (*adapted from Agur, Grant's Atlas 9th Ed, 1991, with permission*).

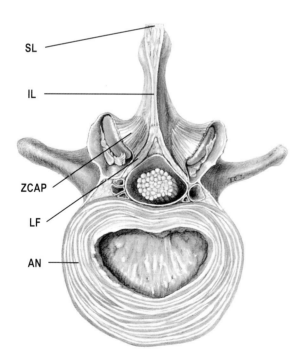

Figure 2.8 Transverse section through a lumbar motion segment - inferior view. SL = supraspinous ligament; IL = interspinous ligament; LF = ligamentum flavum; ZCAP = z-joint capsule; AN = anulus (*adapted from Agur, Grant's Atlas 9th Ed, 1991, with permission*).

terspinous, intertransverse and supraspinous ligaments (figures 2.7 and 2.8). The iliolumbar ligament, a structure which remains controversial in terms of its development and morphology throughout the life span, is found spanning the iliac crest and the transverse process of L5 at the base of the quadratus lumborum muscle (figure 2.9).

As noted above with regard to the intervertebral disc, the lumbar ligaments can be described as having both mechanical and neurological functions. Mechanically, the lumbar ligaments, along with the intervertebral disc, provide a measure of segmental motion control. However, the degree to which these structures mechanically control segmental motion is not as great as was once believed (Oxland & Panjabi, 1992; Panjabi, et al, 1998). While this is discussed in greater detail in the third chapter, it is sufficient at this point to state that the intervertebral disc and ligaments contribute only minimally to the mechanical control of segmental motion.

Individual ligaments are typically believed to control joint movement through a single plane of motion, such as the anterior cruciate ligament controlling anterior translation of the tibia relative to the femur. In reality, most ligaments develop tension through a number of planes of motion. For example, while the anterior longitudinal ligament

(ALL) is ideally suited to assist in the control of end range extension through the lumbar spine, in reality some fibres of the ALL will develop tension as the segment moves through side bending. Other fibres will be tensioned as it moves through rotation. As such, the ALL contributes to segmental motion control in all three planes; one primary and two secondary. When all ligaments acting at a lumbar motion segment are considered, we can expect that a number of ligaments will be involved, to varying degrees, in the control of segmental motion through any single plane of movement.

The neurological function of the lumbar ligaments again involves the provision of proprioceptive sensory feedback to the CNS via the many mechanoreceptors found throughout these structures. These mechanoreceptors play an integral role in the short loop reflex activation of the paraspinal musculature, which is activated when these ligaments are tensioned (Solomonow et al, 1998).

Clinical Application:

When a clinician identifies a single plane of physiological lumbar movement which reproduces the patient's pain, it must be appreciated that a number of osseoligamentous structures are being loaded through that movement. Some will function as primary restraining elements, others in a secondary or even tertiary fashion. In many circumstances, the patient will be painful in more than one plane of movement. As such, identifying the 'single' anatomical structure responsible for the patient's pain is an unrealistic objective.

While the osseoligamentous structures at a lumbar motion segment have a significant role to play in the control of segmental motion, it would appear that this role is primarily neurophysiological. This is of clinical importance as it suggests that if osseoligamentous pathology develops at a lumbar motion segment, the proprioceptive feedback from this segment will be disrupted. This may have negative effects on the neuromuscular control of segmental motion, leading to further load being placed on the injured osseoligamentous structures.

Anatomy of the Deep Segmental Muscles

The muscles with segmental components in the lumbar spine are the psoas major, the quadratus lumborum and the multifidus. Also included in this group is the transversus abdominis. The psoas, quadratus lumborum and multifidus muscles are arranged nearly continuously about the spinal column (figure 2.10), beginning at the anterolateral aspect of the lumbar vertebral body and ending at the lateral aspect of the spinous processes. The following descriptions are based on a dissection conducted by the authors of this text along with our colleague at the University of Toronto, Dr. Anne Agur (Jemmett et al, 2004).

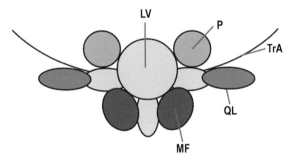

Figure 2.10 Schematic representation of the distribution of deep segmental muscles about a typical lumbar vertebra (LV). P = psoas; TrA = transversus abdominis; QL = quadratus lumborum; MF = multifidus (*modified from Jemmett et al., 2004, with permission*).

Psoas Major

The vertebral attachments of the psoas muscle span the T12-L1 motion segment to the L4-5 intervertebral disc (figure 2.11). Its most cranial elements blend with the crura of the diaphragm. Psoas major is composed of several distinct fascicles (figure 2.13), with each fascicle having a consistent pattern of attachment across a given motion segment. There are two distinct sub-components of each fascicle, a *vertebral* head and a *discal* head.

The most superficial fibres of the vertebral head are continuous with a fibrous arch spanning adjacent superior and inferior vertebral margins (figure 2.12). As fibers of the vertebral head become progressively deeper, they attach along the superior half of the vertebral body, as far posteriorly as the pedicle (figure 2.14). Fibres of the discal head form a broad attachment along the lateral margin of the intervertebral disc from anterior to posterior. The most posterior fibres of the discal head have further and more lateral attachments to the anterior layer of the thoracolumbar fascia and the inferior margin of the transverse process superior to the disc, along its medial two-thirds (figure 2.14). This deepest attachment of the discal head fills the interval between adjacent transverse processes. Distally, each of the fascicles of psoas terminate in a common tendon within the psoas muscle, proximal to its merger with iliacus.

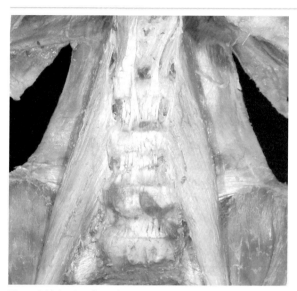

Figure 2.11 Lumbar dissection, anterior view. General relationships between the vertebral column, psoas major and quadratus lumborum.

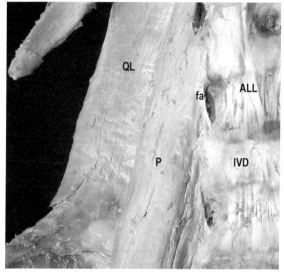

Figure 2.12 Anterior view, right psoas major demonstrating the muscle's anterior and superficial attachments to the anterolateral intervertebral disc (IVD) and fibrous arch (fa). QL = quadratus lumborum; ALL = anterior longitudinal ligament; P = psoas.

Figure 2.13 (left) Anterolateral view, right psoas major - blunt dissection revealing distinct fascicles, each with anterior and superficial attachments to the disc and deeper, more posterior attachments.

Figure 2.14 (below) Anterior view, deep dissection of psoas revealing the attachments of the vertebral (VH) and discal (DH) heads at the L3 vertebral body, the L3-4 intervertebral disc and the L3 transverse process.

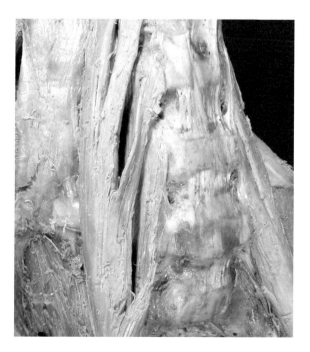

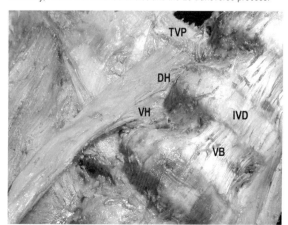

Quadratus Lumborum

The most medial component of the quadratus lumborum spans adjacent transverse processes from L1 to L4 (figure 2.15). Segmentally, these attach along the superolateral third of an inferior transverse process and the inferolateral third of the adjacent superior transverse process. The more lateral components of the quadratus lumborum are multi-segmental. When viewed posteriorly, two distinct patterns of attachment are noted (figure 2.16). The first, between the transverse processes of L1 to L4 and the iliac crest, is somewhat oblique and oriented in an inferolateral direction. The second, between the twelfth rib and the iliac crest, is more vertically oriented. When viewed anteriorly, only the vertically oriented fibres of the lateral component are visible (figure 2.17).

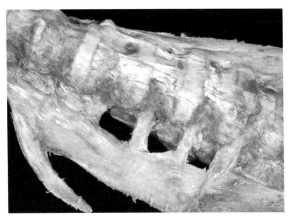

Figure 2.15 Anterolateral view, right quadratus lumborum; all but the most medial fibres run vertically from the 12th rib to the iliac crest.

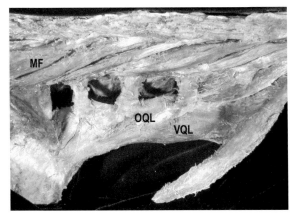

Figure 2.16 Posterolateral view, right quadratus lumborum; bilaminar architecture with oblique fibres (OQL) attaching between the transverse processes of L1 to L4 and the iliac crest and more vertical fibres (VQL) from the 12th rib to the iliac crest. MF = multifidus.

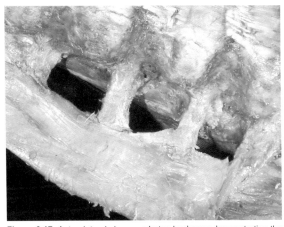

Figure 2.17 Anterolateral view, quadratus lumborum demonstrating the most medial fibres attaching segmentally between lumbar transverse processes.

Multifidus

The lumbar multifidus spans from the S4 to the L1 spinal level (figure 2.18). As with psoas, the multifidus is comprised of several distinct fascicles of varying length and attachment. The general orientation of the muscle varies in both the sagittal and coronal planes from caudal to cranial, with the majority of this variation existing from S4 to L4. In the sagittal plane, fascicles originating from the S4 level maintain a purely axial orientation with subsequently more cranial fascicles becoming progressively more oblique from posterior to anterior.

In the coronal plane, the most caudal fascicles of multifidus originating from the sacrum are essentially vertical. As the sacral component of multifidus becomes more cranial, a more oblique, superomedial fascicular orientation develops with this obliquity becoming maximal at the level of the L5-S1 motion segment. Between the S1 and the L4 level the increase in obliquity plateaus with no further progression beyond the L3 level.

The lumbar multifidus is composed of five distinct fascicles, each inserting at the caudolateral tip of a lumbar spinous process (figure 2.19). The most caudal fascicle, fascicle 5, originates from the posterior surface of the sacrum at the S4 to S3 level and is attached to the L5 spinal level. Fascicle 4 has a broad origin from the posterior sacrum from S3 to the PSIS with its cranial attachment at the L4 spinal level. Fascicle 3 takes its origin from the PSIS and adjacent iliac crest at the S1 spinal level, with its cranial attachment at the L3 spinal level. Fascicle 2 spans the L4-5 motion segment to L2 spinal level. Fascicle 1 originates at the L3-4 motion segment and attaches at the L1 spinal level.

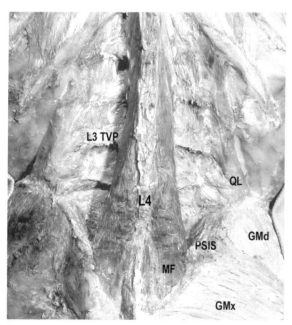

Figure 2.18 Dissection of the deep lumbar region. Prior to blunt or sharp dissection, the lumbar multifidus (MF) appears as a single, large muscle spanning S4 to L1. L4 = position of L4 spinous process. QL = quadratus lumborum; GMx = gluteus maximus; GMd = gluteus medius.

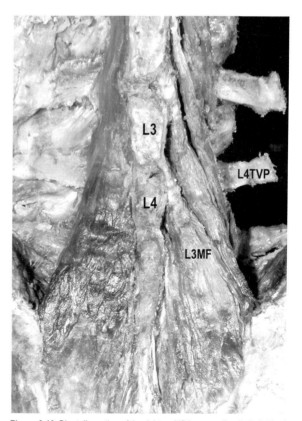

Figure 2.19 Blunt dissection of the right multifidus revealing its individual fasicles. L3 = position of L3 spinous process; L4 = position of L4 spinous process; L3MF = L3 multifidus fasicle.

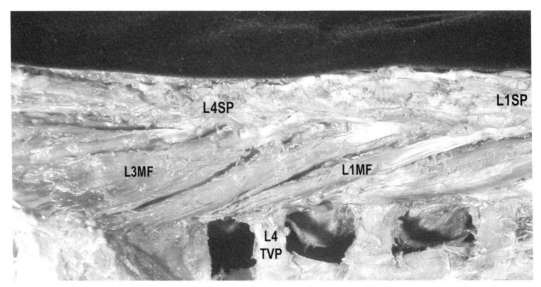

Figure 2.20a Posterolateral view, right side of the lumbar spine and multifidus. Blunt dissection reveals individual fasicles of the multifidus. L4SP = position of L4 spinous process; L1SP = position of L1 spinous process; L4TVP = L4 transverse process; L3MF = L3 fasicle of multifidus; L1MF = L1 fasicle of multifidus.

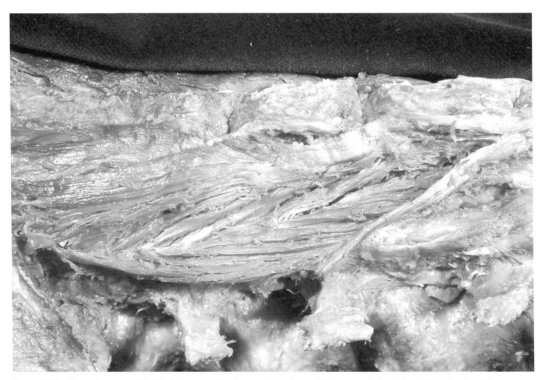

Figure 2.20b Sharp dissecton of fasicle 1 demonstrating the central tendon and bi-pennate design typical of fasicles 1 and 2.

Each fascicle has a fairly complex 'internal' architecture (figure 2.20). The first and second fascicles are each comprised of superficial and deep fibres which arise, bi-pennate style, from a central tendon. The more superficial fibres of each fascicle attach at the tip of a spinous process. The deeper fibres from the same central tendon attach at the base of the spinous process, one level below. The third, fourth and fifth fascicles insert cranially *via* broad attachments from the base to the tip of their respective spinous processes, and caudally along the posterior aspect of the sacrum. Fascicle 3 occupies the largest and most lateral area of insertion and fascicle 5 the smallest and most medial. Laminar fibres also exist at each level, spanning adjacent segments. These deep fibres of multifidus originate at the mamillary process of the more superior vertebra and insert at the z-joint capsule of the more inferior vertebra.

Transversus Abdominis

The lumbar transversus abdominis muscle is fascial anteriorly and posteriorly. Most of its muscular lumbar component is found laterally in the trunk (figure 2.21). In a study of ten cadavers, the posterior transversus abdominis fascia was described as having a direct attachment to the lateral raphe of the thoracolumbar fascia (Bogduk & MacIntosh, 1984). However, this study was limited to a discussion of the muscle's attachments to the posterior and middle layers of the thoracolumbar fascia. Interestingly, our dissection of a single cadaver failed to distinguish any direct attachment of transversus or its fascia to the lateral raphe and thus to the posterior or middle layers of the thoracolumbar fascia. Instead, the transversus abdominis fascia passed anterior to the quadratus lumborum muscle (figures 2.21 and

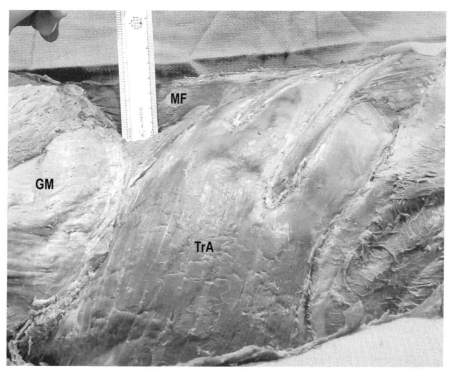

Figure 2.21 Dissection of the lumbar region, right side, lateral view. The external and internal oblique have been reflected demonstrating the transversus abdominis (TrA) muscle and its continuity with the anterior layer of the thoracolumbar fascia. The scale demonstrates the distance between spinous and transverse processes and the depth of the multifidus (MF) muscle at approximately the L4 spinal level. GM = gluteus medius.

24

22) becoming continuous only with the anterior layer of the thoracolumbar fascia (Jemmett et al, 2004). This single layer of fascia covered the protective layer of fat over the kidney and was surprisingly thin and fragile. This inconsistency regarding the posterior attachments of transversus abdominis may represent only a degree of variation in the 'normal anatomy' of this muscle. Conversely, it may be indicative of a need for larger, more comprehensive studies of the muscle's gross anatomy. Figure 2.22 (below) demonstrates the general architectural relationships between the transversus abdominis muscle and other key structures of the lumbar region.

Anatomy of the Superficial Multi-Segmental Muscles

The multi-segmental muscles of the lumbar spine are the longissimus, the iliocostalis, and the rectus abdominis, external oblique and internal oblique.

Longissimus and Iliocostalis

The longissimus and iliocostalis muscles are considered to be two-part muscles with both lumbar and thoracic components acting in the lumbar region. Longissimus pars lumborum arises

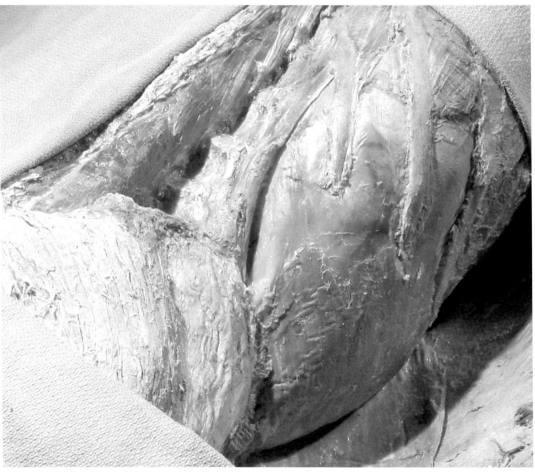

Figure 2.22 Dissection of the lumbar region, right side, posterolateral view. The external and internal oblique have been reflected demonstrating the transversus abdominis and its architectural relationships with the quadratus lumborum and multifidus.

from the lateral half of the posterior aspect of the lumbar transverse processes of L1 to L4, and attaches at an area adjacent to the posterior superior iliac spine of the ilium. The fascicles of L5 attach closer to the posterior inferior iliac spine. Iliocostalis pars lumborum arises from the inferior and posterior tip of the transverse processes of L1 to L4, attaching along the most medial aspect of the iliac crest, along an area bordered by the posterior superior and posterior inferior iliac spines.

Longissimus pars thoracis arises as a tendon from the ribs and thoracic spinous processes from levels T1 to T12. These tendons are three to four centimetres long, with a seven to eight centimetre muscle belly located in the mid-part of the muscle. The caudal end of the muscle is also fascial or tendinous. The muscle attaches in the lumbar region *via* the lumbar spinous processes as well as the sacrum.

Iliocostalis pars thoracis is the most lateral of the erector spinae group, arising from ribs five to twelve. Its most cranial attachment is tendinous with its muscular component found through its mid-length. The muscle attaches caudally *via* a long tendon to the posterior, medial aspect of the iliac crest.

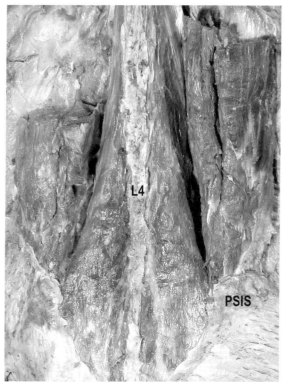

Figure 2.23 Dissection of the lumbar region, posterior view. The three columns of lumbar paraspinal muscle are demonstrated. From medial to lateral are the multifidus, longissimus pars lumborum and the iliocostalis pars lumborum. L4 = position of the L4 spinous process; PSIS = position of the posterior superior iliac spine.

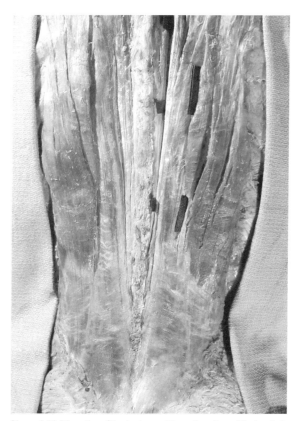

Figure 2.24 Dissection of the lumbar and thoracic regions. The longissimus pars thoracis and the iliocostalis pars thoracis are shown along with their fascial and tendonous attachments to the iliac crest and sacrum.

Rectus Abdominis

Rectus abdominis attaches between the symphysis pubis and the xiphoid process and the 5th to 7th costal cartilages. Its right and left halves are separated by the linea alba, a tendinous structure spanning the xiphoid process to the symphysis pubis. Rectus abdominis is surrounded by the *rectus sheath*, a tough fibrous envelope formed of the right and left abdominal aponeuroses as they approach the anterior midline.

External Oblique

External oblique originates from the anterolateral surfaces of the fifth to twelfth ribs, interdigitating with slips from both the serratus anterior, more superiorly, and the latissimus dorsi, more inferiorly. The fibres of external oblique become aponeurotic prior to inserting to the linea alba, the pubic tubercle and the anterior half of the iliac crest.

Internal Oblique

The internal oblique takes origin from the thoracolumbar fascia, the anterior two thirds of the iliac crest and the lateral two thirds of the inguinal ligament. The thoracolumbar fascial attachments of the muscle are variable and do not develop in all people.

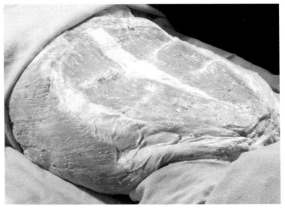

Figure 2.25 Dissection of the anterior and lateral trunk, right side, anterolateral view. The superficial layer of the abdominal aponeurosis has been resected to demonstrate the rectus abdominis and right external oblique.

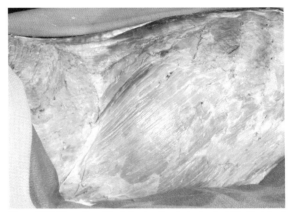

Figure 2.26 Dissection of the lateral and posterior trunk, right side, lateral view. The thoracolumbar fascia and the latissimus dorsi have been resected, demonstrating the external oblique and erector spinae.

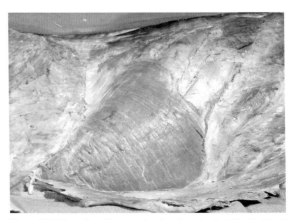

Figure 2.27 Dissection of the lateral and posterior trunk, right side, lateral view. The external oblique has been reflected, demonstrating the internal oblique.

Anatomy of the Thoracolumbar Fascia

The thoracolumbar fascia consists of three layers of fascia which invest and surround the posterior muscles of the lumbar spine (figure 2.28). The *anterior layer* lies anterior to the quadratus lumborum muscle. The *middle layer* is found immediately posterior to quadratus lumborum and thus anterior to the erector spinae group. Both the anterior and middle layers attach to the tips of the lumbar transverse processes.

The *posterior layer* of the thoracolumbar fascia, the most superficial, is formed of two laminae, the superficial and deep laminae (figures 2.29 and 2.30). Located immediately posterior to the multifidus and erector spinae, the two laminae give attachment to a variety of trunk, hip and shoulder muscles. The superficial lamina of the posterior layer is continuous with the caudal aponeurosis of the latissimus dorsi muscle and the external oblique, gluteus medius and gluteus maximus muscles. The deep lamina has similar attachments with the gluteus medius, erector spinae and internal oblique muscles along with the sacrotuberous ligament (Pool-Goudzwaard et al., 1998).

Attachments between the rhomboids and the superficial lamina and between the splenius cervicis and capitus and the deep lamina have also been reported (Barker & Briggs, 1999). In the midline, the posterior layer blends with the supraspinous and interspinous ligaments, forming a continuous musculofascial system with the potential to transmit tensile forces (generated in muscles such as latissimus dorsi, internal oblique and gluteus medius) to the spinal column (Lee, 1999a). The posterior and middle layers of the thoracolumbar fascia have recently been reported to be capable of transmitting tensile forces between the transversus abdominis muscle and the lumbar vertebrae (Barker et al, 2004).

The three layers of the thoracolumbar fascia meet just lateral to the lateral border of the iliocostalis lumborum, forming the dense *lateral raphe*. Bogduk reported that the middle fibres of the transversus abdominis muscle developed from the deep layer of the thoracolumbar fascia *via* the lateral raphe (Bogduk & MacIntosh, 1984).

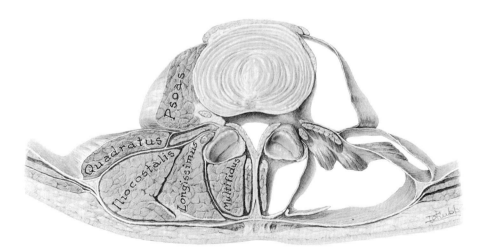

Figure 2.28 Drawing of an superior view of a transverse section through the lumbar region, demonstrating the relationships between the deep lumbar muscles and the thoracolumbar fascia. On the left, the muscles and fascia are in place; on the right the major muscles have been removed (*from Agur, Grant's Atlas, 9th Ed, 1991, with permission*).

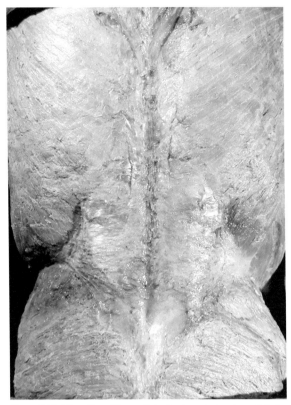

Figure 2.29 Dissection of the posterior trunk, posterior view. Only the skin and sub-cutaneous tissues have been resected, demonstrating the superficial layer including the latissimus dorsi muscles, the posterior layer of the thoracolumbar fascia and the gluteus maximus muscles.

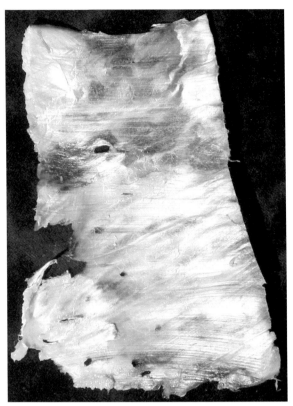

Figure 2.30 The posterior layer of the left thoracolumbar fascia; the midline attachments are on the right side of this photograph. Note the visibly interweaving pattern of the posterior layer's superficial and deep laminae.

Differential Function of the Segmental and Multi-Segmental Muscles

Bergmark (1989) described the muscles of the lumbar region as either *local* or *global*, with local muscles performing a stabilizing role while global muscles were more involved with the generation of movement and the maintenance of overall spinal orientation. We have chosen to use the terms segmental and multi-segmental in place of *local* and *global* to maintain a more consistent terminology throughout this text. Spinal stability has been described as the control of segmental spinal motion via the integrated function of the nervous, muscular and osseoligamentous systems (Panjabi, 1992a). The maintenance of spinal orientation may be described as a function of the neuromuscular system whereby regional vertebral column movements or postures are either produced or maintained.

A more complete discussion of the function of the muscles of the lumbar region is provided in the third chapter. An appreciation for the functional significance of the segmental and multi-segmental muscles requires a more in-depth understanding of segmental biomechanics and current theories of spinal stability. These concepts are developed throughout the remainder of this chapter and throughout the third chapter.

Segmental Biomechanics of the Lumbar Spine

THE CLINICALLY RELEVANT biomechanics of the lumbar region are presented as they have been hypothesized to exist through single directions of movement (e.g., flexion). Each physiological movement is described in terms of its osteokinematics (the motion of a single bone in space, without regard for its behaviour at a specific joint) and in terms of its arthrokinematics (the relative motions of two adjacent vertebrae as they occur at a vertebral motion segment). It should be appreciated that this is a contentious topic, from both the theoretical and applied perspectives.

At present there remains a lack of consensus, among both researchers and clinicians, regarding the theoretical aspects of segmental biomechanics in the lumbar region. This lack of consistent standard involves both the terms used to describe the bone and joint motions as well as the fundamental nature or composition of the motions, most notably in regard to the 'coupled' motion of side bending and axial rotation (Cook, 2003). With regard to physiological flexion and extension, while the terminology might vary between authors, it is agreed that lumbar flexion involves both an anterior sagittal rotation and an anterior translation. Reversely, extension involves a posterior sagittal rotation and a posterior translation. However, despite a number of studies dating back several decades, there is conflicting data describing the patterns of the coupled motions involved in side bending and rotation throughout the lumbar spine (Bogduk, 1997b; Cook, 2003; Cook & Showalter, 2004).

It is generally though not universally agreed that side bending and axial rotation occur together in the lumbar spine. There is reasonable consensus regarding the pattern of coupled motion when rotation is the initiated movement. Most authors report that with initiated rotation, a contralateral side bending occurs from the L1-2 segment to the L3-4 segment and that an ipsilateral side bending occurs at L4-5 and L5-S1 (Pearcy & Tibrewal, 1984; Panjabi et al, 1994: Cholewicki et al, 1996).

However, there is little consensus regarding coupling when the initiated movement is side bending. Utilizing three-dimensional (3-D) measurements of *in-vitro* specimens, Schultz and colleagues and McGlashen and colleagues both reported that coupled motion did not occur when the initial physiological movement was side bending (Schultz et al, 1979; McGlashen et al, 1987). Other 3-D studies have found that the coupling of side bending and rotation can occur, and that in most specimens at most levels, when side bending is the initial movement, the coupled motion is contralateral rotation (Pearcy & Tibrewal, 1984; Panjabi et al, 1989; Cholewicki et al, 1996).

However, there remains a degree of variability even within this 'pattern'. For example, with initial side bending at the L1-2 motion segment, reports of coupled motion vary from none to either ipsilateral or contralateral rotation in some specimens (Panjabi et al, 1989; Panjabi et al, 1994; Cholewicki et al, 1996). Cook, in a review of 3-D coupling experiments, found that on average, most studies reported a contralateral rotation as occurring throughout the remainder of the lumbar spine, that is, from the L2-3 segment to L5-S1 (Cook, 2003). Still, there was some variability, most notably at L4-5 where authors reported either no rotational coupling (McGlashen et al, 1987), ipsilateral coupling (Cholewicki et al, 1996) or contralateral coupling (Panjabi et al, 1994). Of clinical interest is the fact that, despite these inconsistencies, the amount of rotation accompanying side bending is almost negligible, averaging only 1 - 2 degrees at each segment (Pearcy & Tibrewal, 1984).

The lack of consistency with respect to the coupling of side bending and rotation may be partially explained by the fact that different researchers have utilized different imaging techniques in the collection of their data (Cook & Showalter, 2004). Older studies relied on observational or two-dimensional radiographic analyses, both of which are prone to significant errors while more recent investigations utilized a variety of 3-D techniques (Cook, 2003; Cook & Showalter, 2004). It has been suggested that the lack of consensus may in fact represent the true situation - that there is simply a large degree of variation between 'normal' individuals with respect to the pattern of coupled side bending and rotation (Bogduk, 1997c). There may be merit to this argument when we consider that, despite using imaging and investigation techniques similar to those used in lumbar studies, different authors have found that the pattern of coupling in the cervical spine is far more consistent (Mimura et al, 1989; Bogduk & Mercer, 2000). Clinicians who utilize mobilization and manipulative techniques should also be aware of the abject lack of data regarding coupled motions of the lumbar spine in living subjects with spinal pathology who are placed in non-weightbearing, side-lying postures.

Clinical Model of Lumbar Biomechanics

From an applied perspective, the lack of convention regarding lumbar coupling can be a source of confusion for students new to the subject, as well as for clinicians who have studied under one convention or another. This confusion stems from the fact that most manual therapy disciplines are based, at least in part, upon one theory or another regarding the pattern of coupled motions in the lumbar spine. Many of the assessment, mobilization and manipulation techniques utilized in a wide variety of disciplines, including osteopathy, chiropractic and physiotherapeutic manual therapy, are based upon one coupling convention or another. These conventions pertain to the assessment of segmental motion and to the direction of therapeutic mobilizations and manipulations intended to restore more appropriate segmental motion. Coupling theory is also fundamental to the necessary practice of 'locking' the spine prior to the delivery of an effective mobilization or manipulative technique.

The practical implications surrounding the topic of lumbar biomechanics will be explored in greater depth in chapters five and six. For now, for the sake of clarity, the authors have adopted the following convention by which to describe the clinically relevant biomechanics of the lumbar spine. All osteokinematic motions, i.e., the

theoretical movements of an isolated bone, are described as *rotations and translations*. Similarly, arthrokinematic motions, the theoretical movements which occur at a lumbar motion segment, are described using the terms *rock* and *slide*.

As arthrokinematic terms describe *joint* motion, the arthrokinematics for both the interbody joint (the inferior vertebral body, intervertebral disc and superior vertebral body) and both z-joints are detailed. These arthrokinematic descriptions are based on the convention of the more superior vertebra moving in relation to the more inferior vertebra.

Segmental Flexion (figure 2.31a)

Flexion Osteokinematics:
A lumbar vertebra moves through a combination of anterior sagittal translation and anterior sagittal rotation.

Flexion Arthrokinematics:
At the interbody joint, there is a posterior to anterior rock and a posterior to anterior slide. At the bilateral z-joints, there is a superior and anterior slide.

Segmental Extension (figure 2.31b)

Extension Osteokinematics:
A lumbar vertebra moves through a combination of posterior sagittal translation and posterior sagittal rotation.

Extension Arthrokinematics:
At the interbody joint, there is an anterior to posterior rock and an anterior to posterior slide. At the bilateral z-joints, there is an inferior and posterior slide.

Segmental Side Bending (figure 2.31c)

As described previously, the directions and patterns of coupled motions involved with lumbar side bending are contentious and likely highly variable. Furthermore, at only 1 – 2 degrees, the amount of

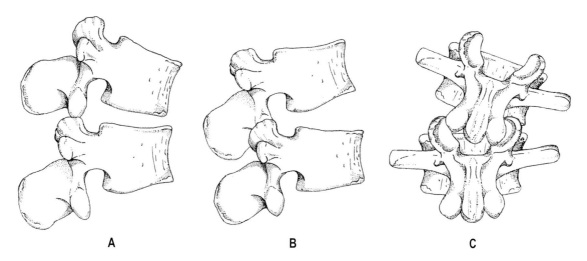

Figure 2.31 Segmental biomechanics of lumbar flexion, extension and sidebending. A - flexion; B - extension; C - right sidebending (modified *from Bogduk, Clinical Anatomy of the Lumbar Spine and Sacrum, 3rd Ed, 1997 with permission*).

rotation may well be clinically insignificant. Therefore the following descriptions do not make reference to any specific pattern of coupled motion which incorporates rotation in the transverse plane.

Side Bending Osteokinematics:
Side bending involves a vertebra moving through an ipsilateral coronal rotation and an ipsilateral coronal translation.

Side Bending Arthrokinematics:
At the interbody joint, an ipsilateral rock and slide in the coronal plane occurs. At the z-joints, unlike the symmetrical motion pattern noted through flexion and extension, an asymmetrical pattern of motion at the right and left z-joints is observed which is dependent on the direction of the physiological spinal movement. For example, with physiological side bending to the right, the right z-joint (the inferior articular process of the superior vertebra) slides inferiorly and medially. The left z-joint (the inferior articular process of the superior vertebra) slides superiorly and medially. During right side bending, the right z-joint is 'compressed' while the left z-joint is 'tensioned'.

Summary

It has been our intention throughout this chapter to review the relevant anatomy of the lumbar region, emphasizing the anatomy of a lumbar motion segment in terms of its passive and active elements, or *subsystems*, and its segmental biomechanics. From a pathoanatomical perspective, the anatomy of the lumbar region might be reviewed with the objective of helping the reader prepare for an examination process aimed at identifying the pathological structure. However, clinical experience and the available literature do not support the ability of the physical examination to consistently and accurately accomplish this goal. Under a segmental dysfunction paradigm, it is more important to prepare clinicians for the task of developing an appreciation for the functional status of the active and passive subsystems acting at a given lumbar motion segment.

As will be discussed in detail in the next chapter, a pattern of deficits affecting a lumbar motion segment may be theorized as being characteristic of most forms of lumbar pathology. Regardless of the pathoanatomical diagnosis, its mode of onset or its severity, the dysfunctional segment will present with an alteration in segmental compliance (i.e., a loss or an increase of intersegmental stiffness) along with an altered pattern of neuromuscular behaviour. The assessment of such deficits is well suited to the skill set of physical therapy.

Orthopaedic physical therapists have a well developed set of manual assessment skills which allow for the clinical assessment of articular and neuromuscular function. Thus, with slight modi-fications in terms of philosophy and test interpretation, it is quite possible for clinicians to develop an accurate and predictable appreciation for the degree of dysfunction affecting a pathologic lumbar motion segment. This, in turn, allows for more effective and predictable management of our patients.

segmental stability & motor control in the lumbar spine

THE TRADITIONAL MODEL of lumbar spine function was based upon the assumption that the non-pathological osseoligamentous spinal column was an inherently stable structure (Knuttson, 1944). This model considered the intervertebral discs, ligaments and osseous elements to be capable of tolerating the loads associated with normal daily activities without need of muscular support (White & Panjabi, 1978). Within this paradigm, a normal spinal radiograph was considered valid evidence of a non-pathological lumbar spinal column. Pathologic spinal *instability* was believed to occur infrequently and secondary only to relatively severe spinal pathology (e.g., spondylolisthesis) or following massive trauma resulting in a significant disruption of the osseoligamentous system.

Recent *in vitro* biomechanical studies have provided evidence challenging these ideas. The spinal loads which develop during daily activities can exceed 6000 N (McGill & Norman, 1986) while certain sports can place loads in excess of 18,000 N through the lumbar spine (Cholewicki et al, 1991). However, studies investigating the load tolerances of the non-muscular spine have demonstrated that the osseoligamentous lumbar or thoracolumbar spine can sustain only 20 to 90

N of load before buckling (Lucas & Bresler, 1961; Crisco et al, 1992). These studies considered the ability of a full region of the spinal column to tolerate loads and maintain a functional posture. Other studies of purely segmental mechanics have found that the disc, ligament, capsular and bony elements of an isolated motion segment can tolerate a maximum load of approximately 65 to 85 N before osseoligamentous pathology develops (Oxland & Panjabi, 1992; Panjabi et al, 1998). Obviously, this dramatic discrepancy between the load bearing capacity of the non-muscular spinal column (both regionally and segmentally) and the loads encountered during normal physical activities does not support the notion that the osseoligamentous lumbar spine is a stable structure. Indeed, the most current evidence reveals that the osseoligamentous lumbar spine is an inherently *unstable* structure (McGill et al, 2003).

This chapter will review the current biomechanical, anatomical and neurophysiological evidence as it relates to the normal and pathological performance of the lumbar spine. This evidence negates the traditional model of lumbar spine function and supports a far more complex yet clinically valid model of spinal behaviour. As will be apparent, this current model accounts for the wide range of patient presentations seen in clinical practice to a far greater extent than does the more traditional pathoanatomical model.

Lumbar Spine Segmental Range of Motion: Physiological ROM, Neutral Zone & Elastic Zone

LUMBAR SEGMENTAL MOTION occurs through the sagittal, coronal and transverse planes of physiological movement (Fryette, 1954; Panjabi, 1998). More recent *in vitro* biomechanical studies have demonstrated that through each of these three planes, the overall physiological spinal ROM may be partitioned into discrete mechanical phases. As these partitions respond quite differently to the onset of osseoligamentous pathology, clinicians must have a sound understanding of these terms and concepts.

Investigations of spinal segmental motion using a progressive physiological loading protocol have identified a consistent pattern of load and deformation in non-pathological lumbar motion segments. When the loads and resultant tissue deformations associated with segmental motion are measured from the so-called *neutral position* (NP) (an *in vitro* motion segment posture in which the loads acting at the segment are minimized) movement of one vertebrae relative to its segmental partner results in a bi-phasic load-deformation curve (Panjabi, 1992a). Based on such data, it has been suggested that the overall physiological range of intervertebral or segmental motion be partitioned into two distinct components. These partitions have been termed the *neutral zone* (NZ) and the *elastic zone* (EZ) (figure 3.1).

Inspection of this load-deformation curve reveals that early in the overall range, the osseoligamentous elements acting at the segment offer little mechanical restraint to segmental motion. This initial partition of the curve, the NZ, is that region of the physiological ROM through

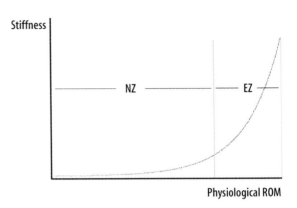

Figure 3.1 Plot of segmental ROM and stiffness (resistance to motion) for a typical lumbar segment demonstrating the bi-phasic nature of segmental motion. The segment experiences little resistance to motion early in range followed by a sharp, non-linear increase in resistance later in range. These phases or partitions of the overall ROM are known as the neutral zone (NZ) and elastic zone (EZ) (*from Jemmett et al, 2004 with permission*).

which segmental motion encounters minimal osseoligamentous stiffness. In clinical terms, we would thus describe the intervertebral disc and ligaments as being unable to provide any appreciable mechanical control of segmental motion through the NZ. The latter phase of the curve, the EZ, represents that component of the physiological ROM in which there is a non-linear increase in the segment's stiffness, or internal resistance to movement. Towards the anatomical limit of the physiological ROM, the osseo-ligamentous elements develop their maximum resistance to segmental motion. However, it is important to recall that the highest loads tolerated by the osseoligamentous elements are likely no more than 80 or 90N. Thus, even at their maximum load bearing capacity, lumbar osseoligamentous structures will be traumatized at loads far below those associated with even 'light' activities of daily living.

While the data reflected in these load-deformation curves are readily captured in the *in vitro* laboratory, the technology does not yet exist to record segmental motion with sufficient resolution to build such a curve using *in vivo* data (Panjabi, 1992b). Nonetheless, the point on the curve at which tension first develops in the osseoligamentous structures, (i.e., the boundary

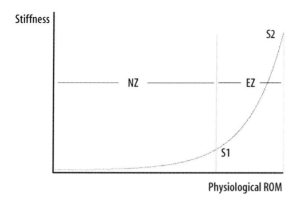

Figure 3.2 Clinical interpretation of the hypothetical NZ:EZ relationship. The boundary between the NZ and EZ is the point at which the clinician appreciates an abrupt increase in the stiffness of the segment (or a decrease in segmental compliance) while the outer limit of the EZ represents the anatomical limit of the segment's available range.

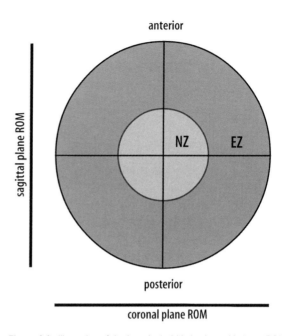

Figure 3.3 Illustration of the hypothetical bi-phasic, multi-planar ROM characteristics typical of lumbar motion segments. This model assumes a symmetrical and equal amplitude for each of the NZ and EZ in each plane of motion (*modified from Jemmett et al., 2004 with permission*).

between the NZ and the EZ), may be appreciated clinically as being the point at which a significant change in segmental stiffness is first noted while performing a passive 'segmental loading or compliance' test (Figure 3.2). As further passive load is applied, stiffness typically increases quickly until a final 'end feel' is noted at the anatomical limit of range.

Although numerous studies have described segmental motion as it occurs through single planes of movement, it is critical for clinicians to appreciate that segmental motion, and thus the NZ and EZ, exist simultaneously in three planes of motion. NZ and EZ motion occurs in anterior and posterior directions in the sagittal plane; in lateral directions in the coronal plane; and in an axial rotation fashion in the transverse plane (figure 3.3). These concepts of *tri-planar segmental motion* provide the foundation for the current model of spinal stability as discussed in the following section.

Stabilization System of the Lumbar Spine

As THE OSSEOLIGAMENTOUS spine is unable to safely contend with normal physiological loads, spinal motion segments are dependent primarily on muscle for their architectural integrity or stability. The current literature supports the hypothesis that this segmental stability is maintained by the spinal muscles *via* the development of adequate intervertebral stiffness. Given the dynamic nature of spinal segmental biomechanics, it is necessary for spinal muscles to be precisely controlled by the central nervous system in order to meet the stability challenges inherent in functional activities. Therefore, it has been proposed that stability of the spinal column is maintained through the integrated function of a three-part, spinal stabilization system comprised of the active (muscular), passive (bony, disc, fascial and ligament) and neural control *subsystems* (figure 3.4) (Panjabi, 1992a). Working independently of Panjabi, Vleeming and colleagues have suggested a similar scheme to explain the stability mechanisms acting at the pelvis (Vleeming et al, 1995). Their integrated model of 'form and force closure' (Pool-Goudzwaard et al, 1998) is

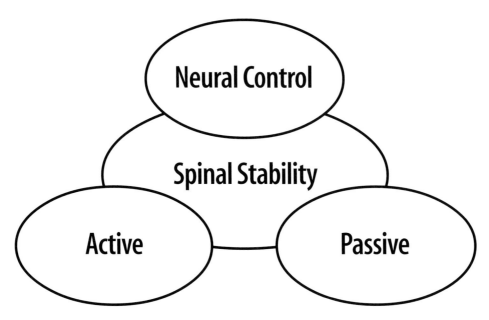

Figure 3.4 Spinal stabilization model as proposed originally by Panjabi. The maintenance of spinal stability is an integrated function of the neural control subsystem, the active subsystem and the passive subsystem (*adapted from Panjabi, 1992a*).

analogous to Panjabi's passive, active and neural control subsystems model. The following is an overview of the components of each of the stabilization subsystems, along with a discussion of the mechanisms by which each contributes to spinal stability.

The Passive Subsystem

THE PASSIVE SUBSYSTEM is composed of the osseoligamentous elements of a lumbar motion segment (the osseous and articular structures, discs, ligaments, and the passive elements of muscle) and has both mechanical and neurological functions. From a mechanical perspective, as seen in the load-deformation curves described previously, the passive subsystem develops little stiffness throughout the tri-planar NZ. The osseo-ligamentous elements of a lumbar motion segment develop tension, and thus stiffness, only towards the end of the physiological range, throughout the tri-planar EZ. Given the low load tolerance of an osseoligamentous lumbar motion segment, this EZ stiffness contributes only minimally to the functional stability of the lumbar spine. Neurologically, the passive subsystem is involved in providing proprioceptive feedback to the central nervous system (CNS) via various mechano- receptors in the intervertebral disc, spinal ligaments and the z-joint capsules. There is growing evidence that this proprioceptive feedback is triggered by tension in the passive subsystem, moreso than with elongation of its tissues (Solomonow et al, 1999).

The Active Subsystem

THE ACTIVE SUBSYSTEM is comprised of segmental and multi-segmental spinal muscles and, like the passive subsystem, has both mechanical and neurological functions. Neurologically, the active subsystem provides proprioceptive feedback to the neural control subsystem *via* its muscle spindles and golgi tendon organs. Mechanically, the active subsystem maintains the functional orientation of the lumbar region and generates sufficient stiffness at individual motion segments to provide adequate segmental stability. Importantly, the active subsystem must be capable of maintaining regional postures and segmental stability without developing undue rigidity throughout the trunk (Hodges, 2004).

As was discussed in the preceding section, the passive subsystem contributes to the mechanical control of segmental motion towards the end of the physiological range, although minimally. Thus, from a mechanical perspective, the active subsystem is solely responsible for generating the intervertebral stiffness required to maintain stability through the tri-planar NZ, and primarily responsible for ensuring stability towards the end of range through the tri-planar EZ. The active subsystem is responsible for the dissipation of spinal loads such that the forces that do reach the osseoligamentous elements are within tolerable limits.

The Neural Control Subsystem

THE NEURAL CONTROL SUBSYSTEM is comprised of the neural components of the active and passive subsystems, their connections to the CNS, and the CNS centers of motor planning and initiation. The nervous system is a critical component of the stabilizing system of the spine, given the absolute need for spinal muscle to provide dynamic control of the relatively unstable osseoligamentous spinal column (Cholewicki, 2003). The proprioceptive information generated by the mechanoreceptors located throughout the active and passive subsystems is utilized by the CNS as a dynamic basis for feedforward motor planning, and as part of a feedback mechanism to monitor the results of previously initiated motor commands. Deficits in the passive subsystem will certainly impair the ability of the CNS to coordinate the active subsystem. The neural control subsystem's task of anticipating and interpreting the dynamic stability needs of the lumbar spine and correctly

activating the active sub-system in order to maintain regional postures and segmental stability is enormously complex (Panjabi, 1992a). Arguably, the physiotherapeutic interventions discussed in chapter six have their greatest therapeutic effect through the neural control subsystem.

Stabilization of the Lumbar Spine in Non-Pathologic Populations: Anatomical, Biomechanical & Neurophysiological Evidence

The preceding sections reviewed the theoretical basis for an integrated, three-part lumbar stabilization system. This section reviews the current evidence regarding the actual mechanisms by which stabilization of the lumbar spine is maintained in normal populations.

THE POTENTIAL FOR VARIOUS SEGMENTAL and multi-segmental muscles of the trunk to stabilize the lumbar spine has been investigated (Panjabi et al, 1989; Wilke et al, 1995; Cholewicki & McGill, 1996; Cholewicki et al, 1997; Quint et al, 1998; Stokes & Gardner-Morse, 2003; Hodges et al, 2003). While all trunk muscles have some capacity to stabilize the lumbar spine, the segmental muscles have unique advantages in this regard. Segmental muscles are capable of providing functional intervertebral stiffness at a lumbar motion segment (Panjabi et al, 1989; Bergmark, 1989; Quint et al, 1998) without the production of secondary torques (Hodges & Moseley, 2003). Thus, segmental muscles can provide control over segmental motion without excessively limiting segmental movement. It is reasonable to expect that during relatively low load activities the multi-segmental muscles will be activated to a lesser extent than during high load sport and occupational activities. Clinically, it seems that it should not be necessary for the multi-segmental muscles to be as active while walking or getting out of a car as when lifting something very heavy.

An activity specific balance between trunk rigidity and segmental stability is necessary for optimal spinal function.

Various terms have been developed to describe the muscles comprising the active subsystem. The terms *local* and *global* have been suggested (Bergmark, 1989) as have *inner* and *outer unit* (Lee, 1999b) to differentiate between muscles which control segmental motion and those which maintain the orientation of the lumbar region. We have adopted the terms *segmental stabilizing muscle* (SSM) and *multi-segmental postural muscle* (MPM) in an effort to best represent the relationships between structure and function with respect to these muscles.

Lumbar muscles with the potential to increase segmental stiffness and thus stabilize segmental motion have been identified through a variety of research approaches. Anatomical and architectural investigations (Macintosh & Bogduk, 1986; Macintosh et al, 1986; Macintosh & Bogduk, 1987; Macintosh & Bogduk, 1991; Gibbons, 2001; Jemmett et al, 2004), *in vitro* biomechanical studies (Crisco & Panjabi, 1991; Kaigle et al, 1995; Quint et al, 1998; Wilke et al, 2003), postural perturbation studies using surface and fine wire electromyography (Hodges & Richardson, 1996; Moseley et al, 2002) and biomechanical modeling (McGill & Norman, 1986; Cholewicki & McGill, 1996) have all been employed in an effort to determine which muscles provide stability in the lumbar spine.

Upon review of this large body of research, there is compelling evidence supporting the suggestion that four lumbar muscles, the multifidus, quadratus lumborum, psoas and transversus abdominis, function as segmental stabilizing muscles. As reviewed in chapter two, each of these muscles has a segmental pattern of attachment in the lumbar spine. As a group, these muscles are distributed around the lumbar spinal column in a manner very suitable to the control of tri-planar segmental motion (figure 3.5) (Jemmett et al, 2004). Thus, from an architectural perspective, there is good evidence supporting their proposed function as segmental stabilizers. From a neurophysiological perspective, there is evidence supportive of the proposal that two of these muscles, the multifidus and the transversus abdominis, are utilized by the neural control subsystem to provide 'fine tuning' and control of segmental motion.

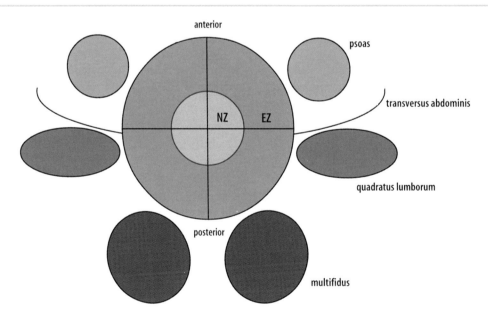

Figure 3.5 Illustration of the architectural relationships between the psoas, quadratus lumborum, multifidus and transversus abdominis muscles superimposed over the hypothetical neutral zone:elastic zone model (NZ, neutral zone; EZ, elastic zone) (*modified from Jemmett et al., 2004, with permission*).

Electromyograhpic studies of multifidus and transversus abdominis using both human and animal subjects have been reported. In human studies of feedforward trunk muscle activation patterns in the setting of a postural perturbation (*via* a rapid movement of the upper or lower extremity), the transversus abdominis is consistently activated prior to the prime mover and in a non-direction specific manner (Hodges & Richardson, 1996; Hodges & Richardson, 1997b; Hodges et al, 1999; Moseley et al, 2002). That is, the transversus abdominis is activated in advance of the prime mover regardless of whether there is a flexion, abduction or extension moment generated *via* limb movement.

Similar electromyographic studies focusing on the multifidus muscle have been performed (Moseley et al, 2002; Moseley et al, 2003). Moseley and colleagues reported that the deep and superficial fibres of the lumbar multifidus were differentially active in subjects without a history of low back pain. Their study found that while the superficial fibers were recruited in a direction-specific fashion, the deep fibers were active in a non-direction specific pattern, similar to that recorded in transversus abdominis (Moseley et al, 2002). This differential activation was further supported by a study which evaluated the effect of expected and unexpected trunk loading on the activation of the deep and superficial fibres of the lumbar multifidus. There was an increase in baseline activity in the deep multifidus prior to the initiation of trunk loading which was not observed in the superficial multifidus (Moseley et al, 2003). Both provide evidence that the neural control subsystem may utilize the deep multifidus to generate a protective measure of segmental stiffness. Further research in this area is certainly required.

Multi-segmental trunk muscles such as the rectus abdominis, external oblique and the lumbar erector spinae are activated in a variable, yet still predictable fashion during a postural perturbation task. These 'direction-specific' muscles activate earlier when required to maintain the orientation of the trunk and later when not required for this purpose. For example, movement of the shoulder into flexion will induce an anterior shift of the center of mass. In preparation, the erector spinae will activate 15 to 21 milliseconds (ms) prior to the deltoid to counter this potential displacement of the trunk into flexion (Hodges et al, 1999). However, if the task requires extension of the shoulder, the upcoming extension moment cannot be countered by the erector spinae and thus it activates 70 to 100 ms after the deltoid (Hodges et al, 1999). In this instance, rather than the erector spinae being active early in anticipation of the upcoming postural challenge, the external oblique would activate early in order to maintain the neutral orientation of the trunk. Interestingly, Moseley and colleagues showed that the superficial fibers of multifidus are recruited in a similar manner, mimicking the activation pattern of the erector spinae (Moseley et al, 2002).

In addition to anticipatory, feedforward mechanisms, the neural control subsystem appears to utilize proprioceptive feedback in its recruitment of muscles such as multifidus. Using an animal model, Solomonow and colleagues investigated the relationship between tensioning of the lumbar supraspinous ligament and activation of the lumbar multifidus (Solomonow et al, 1998). It was shown that with a passive stretch of the supraspinous ligament sufficient to create flexion of the lumbar spine (and thus deformation of the L4-5 disc as well as the motion segments above and below the L4-5 level), the multifidus adjacent to the moving segments was activated. The degree of segmental multifidus activation was in relation to the degree of passive segmental flexion, and thus the tensioning of the passive elements at each segment.

To date, neither quadratus lumborum nor psoas has been studied using EMG during a postural perturbation protocol. While some studies of the recruitment of quadratus lumborum during a variety of activities and conditioning exercises have been reported (Andersson et al, 1996; McGill et al, 1996), such studies shed little light on the strategies employed by the neural control subsystem specific to the generation of segmental stiffness and spinal stability.

42

Summary

Presently, there is good multi-disciplinary evidence to support the following hypotheses regarding the maintenance of spinal stability in non-pathologic populations:

1. Spinal stability is a function of the integrated behavior of the passive, active and neural control subsystems.

2. The objectives of this stabilizing system are:

   i) the generation of intersegmental stiffness and the dissipation of spinal loads such that the functionally fragile osseoligamentous spine is not injured and,

   ii) the utilization of the segmental and multi-segmental muscles in an activity-specific manner ensuring an optimal balance between rigidity and mobility, both segmentally and regionally.

3. The neural control subsystem utilizes both feedforward and feedback mechanisms to optimally coordinate the various segmental muscles of the active subsystem.

4. The segmental muscles most likely to generate intersegmental stiffness and thus control tri-planar segmental motion are the transversus abdominis, psoas, quadratus lumborum and the multifidus.

Stabilization of the Lumbar Spine in Pathologic Populations: Biomechanical, Anatomical & Neurophysiological Evidence

Lumbar Pathology & Segmental Biomechanics

IN VITRO STUDIES OF THE LOAD bearing capacity of individual spinal motion segments have been reported (Oxland & Panjabi, 1992; Panjabi et al, 1998). Such studies subject fresh cadaveric osseoligamentous motion segments to progressive simulated physiological loads until failure (i.e., pathology) occurs in some component of the osseoligamentous spine. At failure, which typically occurred at loads no higher than 9 kg or 90N, the types of injuries sustained included the full range of potential traumatic osseoligamentous pathology: vertebral rim and/or endplate fractures, ligament avulsions and sprains, along with a variety of disc and z-joint lesions, were reported (Oxland & Panjabi, 1992).

As these passive subsystem lesions developed, the amplitude of the NZ consistently increased. This is not an unexpected outcome since the boundary between the NZ and the EZ is defined as the point in range at which significant tension begins to develop in the passive structures. If a passive structure becomes pathological, if it is stretched, torn or otherwise damaged, it will not develop its normal tension or stiffness until some further point in the range. Thus, as traumatic pathology develops within the passive subsystem, the boundary between the NZ and EZ shifts and the amplitude or size of the tri-planar NZ is increased (figure 3.6).

Similar changes in the presence of degenerative disc disease have been reported. Salter described segmental instability as a pattern of uneven, excessive segmental motion resulting from degenerative changes in the lumbar spine (Salter, 1999). In a series of reports in the mid 1980's, Gertzbein and colleagues investigated the

anterior

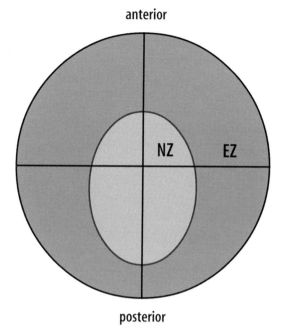

posterior

Figure 3.6 The bi-phasic, multi-planar ROM characteristics hypothesized to be typical of pathologic lumbar motion segments. With the onset of osseoligamentous pathology, NZ amplitude is markedly increased relative to EZ amplitude and overall ROM; in this example, pathology has resulted in a larger NZ, primarily in the sagittal plane and in the posterior direction (*modified from Jemmett et al., 2004, with permission*).

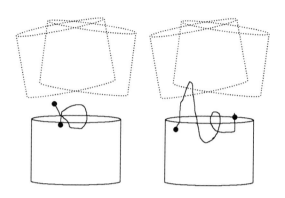

Figure 3.7 As a spinal segment moves through range, its axis of rotation varies - when the path of this rotational axis is plotted throughout range it is known as a centrode. As shown on the left, healthy lumbar motion segments generate tightly clustered centrodes. As shown on the right, lumbar motion segments with mild to moderate degenerative changes develop more chaotic centrodes, suggestive of poorly controlled motion (*based on Gertzbein et al., 1985*).

quality and pattern of lumbar segmental motion in degenerative disc disease (Gertzbein et al, 1985; Gertzbein et al, 1986). Using the path of the instantaneous axis of rotation (PIAR) as a marker of segmental stability and motion quality, they found that lumbar motion segments with even minor degenerative changes displayed a larger and more chaotic PIAR than did the non-pathological motion segments (figure 3.7). These findings, in the setting of mild to moderate degenerative changes, fit well with those described above with regard to increased NZ amplitudes in traumatically induced pathology. Conversely, severe degenerative changes with osteophyte formation may be expected to increase segmental stiffness and thus limit NZ motion (Panjabi, 1992a).

There is now good evidence supporting the assertion that changes in the size of the NZ represent the single most sensitive indicator of the presence of pathology in the osseoligamentous lumbar spine. With most forms of passive subsystem pathology, the amplitude of the NZ increases dramatically while the overall ROM increases only minimally; the typical NZ:ROM ratios determined experimentally range from approximately 6:1 to as high as 17:1 (Panjabi et al, 1998). This significant finding predicts much of what is commonly seen in clinical practice. For example, radiographs are rarely helpful in diagnosing the primary lesion in patients with low back pain. Since current imaging technologies are unable to detect changes in the amplitude of the NZ, it is anticipated that many instances of osseoligamentous pathology will continue to go undetected. From an etiological perspective, the fact that such pathology develops secondary to loads far below those associated with ADLs is more predictive of the typical mechanism of injury reported by many patients.

Anatomical Changes in the Presence of Lumbar Pathology

IN THE PRESENCE OF BOTH acute and chronic lumbar pathology, various histological and gross anatomical changes occur in the lumbar multifidus muscle. Microscopy, ultrasound, CT and MR imaging studies have identified decreased cross sectional area (Hides et al, 1994; Barker et al, 2004), increased intramuscular fat relative to healthy muscle tissue (Parkkola et al, 1993; Kader et al, 2000) and degenerative changes in type I as well a selective atrophy of type II muscle fibres in the lumbar multifidus (Rantanen et al, 1993). Some of these changes have been specific to the clinically determined level of dysfunction (Hides et al, 1994) or at the level of intervertebral disc prolapse (Zhao et al, 2000; Yoshihara et al, 2001). In a recent study of patients with unilateral low back pain (Barker et al, 2004), the loss of cross sectional area (CSA) was greatest (21.1% – 21.6%) at the clinically determined level of dysfunction; however, multifidus CSA was also reduced one level above and below this primary dysfunctional level, although to a lesser extent (15.2% - 18.2%). The exact mechanism underlying these histological and anatomical changes remains uncertain. Reflex inhibition, impaired proprioception, muscle protein breakdown secondary to inflammation and alterations in local circulation are all potential causes for these changes. Further research is required.

Alterations in the anatomical and physiological CSA of the lumbar multifidus can persist following the resolution of symptoms and in the presence of chronic or recurrent low back pain. In a study of patients with acute-onset, first-episode low back pain, Hides and colleagues reported a segmental loss of multifidus volume which persisted beyond resolution of the subject's symptoms (Hides et al, 1996). In a study in which patients were followed for five years following discectomy, muscle biopsies taken at surgery and at five year follow-up showed that the type 1 muscle fibres taken from a sample of the multifidus muscle, at the pathological spinal level, demonstrated a physiological decrease in cross sectional area (Rantanen et al, 1993).

Other studies have found evidence of severe histological deficits in the multifidus muscle in the presence of degenerative spondylolisthesis (Ramsbacher et al, 2001), following retraction during spinal surgery (Taylor et al, 2002) and in patients with intervertebral disc herniation (Zhao et al, 2000; Yoshihara et al, 2001). While the loss of physiological multifidus volume (i.e., a reduction in muscle fibre diameter rather than whole muscle CSA) has been reported as occurring both unilaterally (Yoshihara et al, 2001) and bilaterally (Sihvonen et al, 1993), it is interesting to note that in most cases, patients with only a unilateral loss of physiological volume had either unilateral symptoms and/or pathology (e.g., disc herniation), whereas those patients with bilateral loss of physiological volume had bilateral, and potentially more severe dysfunction (e.g., a laminectomy). Segmental losses of CSA have also been reported in the psoas muscle ipsilateral to an intervertebral disc herniation (Dangaria & Naesh, 1998) as well as in patients with unilateral 'non-specific' low back pain (Barker et al, 2004).

Altered Motor Control in the Presence of Lumbar Pathology

A NUMBER OF STUDIES have found evidence suggestive of altered motor function in the muscles of the lumbar spine in the presence of low back pain (Hodges & Richardson, 1996; Radebold et al, 2000; Hodges 2001; Marras et al, 2001; Radebold et al, 2001; van Dieen et al, 2003; Fergusson et al, 2004; Ferreira et al, 2004; MacDonald et al, 2004; Silfies et al, *in press*). In two EMG-based postural challenge studies of patients with chronic low back pain, activation of the transversus abdominis was altered (Hodges & Richardson, 1996; Hodges & Richardson, 1998). The transversus abdominis was significantly delayed, activating after the prime mover in trials where rapid movements of upper or lower limbs were used to induce perturbations to the spine. Interestingly, this delayed activation differed depending on the direction of the limb movement. The transversus abdominis became delayed and direction specific, demonstrating a pattern of activation similar to that of the superficial, multi-segmental abdominal muscles. In a recent study, the degree of activation of the transversus abdominis, internal oblique and external oblique were measured in subjects with recurrent low back pain during a task involving lower limb motion from a supine posture. The internal and external oblique activations were unchanged relative to controls while activity in the transversus abdominis was reduced in the low back pain group (Ferreira et al, 2004). It has been proposed that the normal *feedforward* activation of transversus abdominis is somehow altered due to the presence of painful stimuli from the lumbar spine (Hodges & Moseley, 2003).

Marras and colleagues, in a study of patients with a range of symptomatic histories, reported on the motor control patterns and spinal loads associated with lifting. Patients demonstrated significantly increased muscle activation along with significantly increased spinal load and segmental motion, in the form of lateral shear (Marras et al, 2001). A greater reliance on co-activation strategies, with a diminished utilization of context specific motor patterning, has also been reported in low back pain populations (Radebold et al, 2000; Marras et al, 2001). In a study comparing motor control strategies during lifting activities in low back pain patients and asymptomatic controls, Ferguson and colleagues found that the erector spinae muscles were active earlier and longer in the low back pain group. They argued that this altered motor control strategy would expose this population to higher spine loads and increase their risk of progressive spinal pathology (Ferguson et al, 2004).

The human lumbar multifidus has been studied extensively in terms of its gross and histological changes in the presence of lumbar pathology; however, little direct study of its neurophysiological behavior in patients with low back pain has been conducted. While we acknowledge that the anatomical changes discussed earlier may develop secondary to a number of mechanisms, altered motor control should be considered a reasonable culprit. Hides and colleagues demonstrated a segmental loss of multifidus volume, ipsilateral to the symptomatic side in a group of patients with recent onset, first-time low back pain. The development of this loss of volume was reported to have occurred as quickly as twenty four hours following the onset of pain (Hides et al, 1994). Such a rapid change implies a neurologically mediated process and is in accordance with similar findings in muscles local to peripheral joints with induced or simulated pathology (Spencer et al, 1984).

To date, only one study has directly considered the neurophysiological behaviour of the deep and superficial fibres of the multifidus muscle in patients with low back pain. MacDonald and colleagues, using a postural perturbation protocol, found evidence of altered recruitment of the deep fibers of multifidus in patients with a history of unilateral low back pain (MacDonald et al, 2004). In subjects with low back pain, the deep multifidus was delayed relative to controls during both flexion and extension of the arm. Further, the differential activation of DM and SM was lost on the symptomatic side (MacDonald et al, 2004).

As described earlier, Solomonow and colleagues developed an *in vivo* feline model to study the relationship between passive stretching of the supraspinous ligament (i.e., passive elements) and activation of the lumbar multifidus (Solomonow et al, 1998). Again, it was shown that with tensioning of the passive elements during flexion of the lumbar spine the lumbar multifidus muscle adjacent to the flexing segments was activated. In a subsequent study, the same feline model was exposed to fifty minutes of continuous cyclic stretching of the supraspinous ligament (Solomonow et al, 1999). Each passive stretch cycle lasted four seconds. As in the 1998 study, the initial stretch cycles of the passive elements resulted in a reflexive activation of the multifidus muscle. However, following eight minutes of continuous cyclic stretching of the supraspinous ligament, multifidus activation was reduced to only 15% of its initial value. By the fifty minute mark, multifidus activation had diminished even further, to as little as 5% of its initial value. The investigators were able to demonstrate that this loss of reflexive multifidus activation was secondary to the development of creep within the passive elements. With further tensioning of the supraspinous ligament sufficient to account for creep, the multifidus activation was restored to normal levels.

The findings of the Solomonow study correlate well with the biomechanical and anatomical research discussed thus far. It is reasonable to expect that the creep which developed within the passive subsystem would have led to an increased NZ at the involved segment. As this occurred, the multifidus muscle local to the now mechanically unstable segment experienced a significant degree of motor impairment. When the creep effect was abolished, the observed motor impairment immediately resolved. It should be noted that by re-tensioning the supraspinous ligament to correct for the effects of creep, the amplitude of the NZ was not restored to normal. Rather, the normal tension characteristics of the ligament were re-established. This may have had the effect of restoring the proprioceptive feedback from the supraspinous ligament and its resultant activation of the adjacent multifidus.

Interpretation of Motor Control Changes in the Presence of Lumbar Dysfunction

"We do not see things as they are, we see them as we are" ..... Anais Nin

NOT SURPRISINGLY, there are conflicting interpretive opinions within the research community regarding the motor control alterations seen in patients with low back pain. While there is agreement that patients with low back pain differ from healthy people in terms of spinal motor control, there is disagreement as to whether this altered motor control represents an adaptive or maladaptive response. Recently, a series of articles was published in the *Journal of Electromyography and Kinesiology*, summarizing the current evidence regarding the key mechanisms surrounding lumbar dysfunction. The editors of this series (Cholewicki et al, 2003) commented on this lack of consensus:

"... the same changes in motor control can be interpreted as functional or dysfunctional depending on the point of view. For example, van Dieen et al and Hodges and Moseley performed extensive literature reviews. Both groups concluded that muscle activation patterns in low back pain populations are not consistent with either the pain-spasm-pain nor pain–adaptation models proposed in the past. However, while van Dieen et al emphasized possible functional adaptations by pointing out positive effects of altered muscle recruitment patterns, Hodges and Moseley emphasized dysfunction by outlining the deleterious effects of such changes."

While intellectually stimulating, such controversies are understandably a source of frustration for clinicians under increasing pressure to base their patient management decisions on the scientific literature. The lack of consensus regarding the functional or dysfunctional nature of these motor control changes is significant as these apparently opposing interpretations logically lead to two very different models of therapeutic intervention (figure 3.8). One clinical model emphasizes the facilitation of an independent activation of the transversus abdominis and multifidus muscles from the superficial trunk flexors and extensors while the other focuses on training or conditioning the multi-segmental muscles of the trunk using exercises such as lateral bridging or contralateral shoulder and hip extension from a quadruped position. To some extent, the controversy regarding motor control is likely influenced by a more fundamental lack of concurrence regarding the larger issue of spinal stability itself.

From an engineering perspective, stability may be conceptualized as the ability of the spine to tolerate the loads imposed upon it during daily activities. Biomechanical engineering often describes the stability of a structure in Eulerian terms, the stability of the structure being directly related to its stiffness. By extension, this implies that increased stiffness equates with improved or more optimal stability. *In vitro* biomechanical studies have shown that segmental as well as multi-segmental muscles can increase segmental stiffness

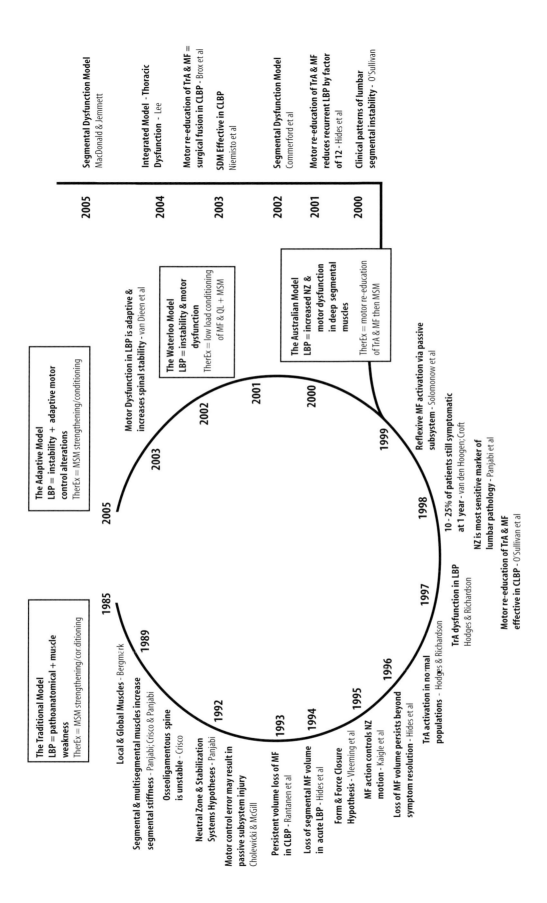

Figure 3.8 The literature regarding the motor control changes associated with lumbar pathology has led to two competing interpretations, the 'adaptive' and the 'maladaptive' models. Each logically leads to its own model of clinical intervention.

(Panjabi et al, 1989; Crisco & Panjabi, 1991). Regarding altered motor control in low back pain, the adaptive interpretation is based on the observation that patients utilize a wide variety of motor control strategies in order to maintain lumbar stability (van Dieen, 2003b). In general, and although the precise tactics vary from patient to patient, there is evidence that the neural control subsystem increases the activation of the multi-segmental muscles in presence of lumbar dysfunction (Marras et al, 2001; Ferguson et al, 2004). Assuming that increased stiffness equates positively with improved stability, and given that multi-segmental muscles can increase segmental stiffness, the strategy of compensating with the multi-segmental muscles appears to be a viable and effective means of maintaining a stable spine. Indeed, in the initial stages following the onset of symptoms, this is likely a very functional strategy.

While an increased utilization of the multi-segmental muscles may be necessary in the short term, there appear to be costs associated with the maintenance of this strategy in the long term. Although biomechanical models have estimated that the paraspinal muscles might restore stability to the lumbar spine at activation levels as low as 1 – 3% (Cholewicki & McGill, 1996) other studies have found that patients with low back pain excessively activate their multi-segmental muscles during functional tasks (Marras et al, 2001; Ferguson et al, 2004; Silfies et al, *in press*). Similar studies have found that patients typically utilize co-contraction strategies involving the multi-segmental muscles to maintain stability (Radebold et al, 2000). It has been argued that the increased spinal loads and compromised respiratory function observed in patients with low back pain are a result of these compensatory strategies (Marras et al, 2001; Ferguson et al, 2004; Hodges, 2004).

Although the alterations in motor control in patients with low back pain might be appreciated as being functional or adaptive in the period immediately following the onset of symptoms, any interpretation of this as an efficient or effective strategy over the longer term is unsupportable for two primary reasons. First, simply increasing spinal stiffness does not equate with optimal stability

in all situations. Increases in the stiffness of the trunk *via* the action of the multi-segmental muscles will, at some point, move beyond optimal stability and be better described as rigidity where the patient loses necessary mobility. Second, based upon epidemiological studies, the strategy is not especially effective beyond the acute stage of recovery.

Whereas an engineer might equate increased trunk rigidity with more optimal spinal stability, the clinician recognizes this rigidity as the typical pathological pattern with which most low back pain patients present. It is not at all unusual to see patients who have adopted a rigidity strategy for walking or rolling out of bed that would be more appropriately reserved for lifting some significant amount of weight from an awkward posture. Optimal spinal stability is a dynamic construct requiring an activity appropriate balance between intersegmental stiffness and the maintenance of regional postures while allowing for an adequate freedom of motion, both segmentally and regionally, so as to permit functional, painfree movement.

The analogy of the flexible pole supported by guy wires to illustrate the concept of stiffness and stability is common (McGill, 2002a). The guy wires add stiffness to the pole and are often used to demonstrate the stability-enhancing functions of the multi-segmental muscles (figure 3.9).

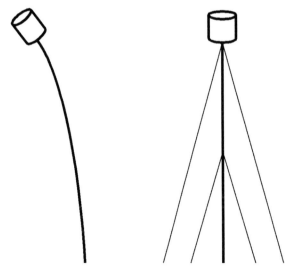

Figure 3.9 The flexible column gives way under loads which exceed its stiffness capacity. Supporting the column with guy wires effectively increases the column's stiffness and thus its load bearing capacity.

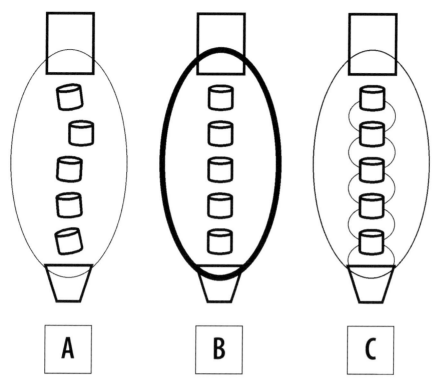

Figure 3.10 Extending the flexible column analogy to the *in vivo* spine requires the addition of short segmental muscles stabilizing each motion segment. **A** - at physiologically and biomechanically optimal recruitment levels, the long multi-segmental muscles (guy wires) are unable to generate sufficient stiffness to stabilize individual motion segments. **B** - the long multi-segmental muscles, if activated to higher than normal levels, can create sufficient stiffness throughout the trunk to achieve control of segmental motion; however, the costs associated with such a strategy are problematic. **C** - a task-appropriate degree of co-contraction amongst the segmental and multi-segmental muscles provides optimal segmental stability while allowing for necessary spinal mobility.

A significant omission in this analogy is the fact that the human spine is not a single flexible rod but a series of inflexible rods (vertebrae) lightly held together by highly elastic 'joiners' (intervertebral discs and ligaments). A more accurate representation would include the need for sets of short guy wires reinforcing each joiner to maintain stability at each 'segment' (figure 3.10). Such a model allows for the competing but necessary demands of stability and mobility in the functional human spinal column.

As stated in Chapter 1, the utility of any model is dependent on the degree to which it predicts events in the real world. Thus, we can assess the adaptive interpretation itself, as well as the clinical models which derive from it, on the basis of clinical efficacy: if the motor control changes observed in patients with low back pain are adaptive, to what extent is this strategy effective in achieving effective spinal stability and a lasting relief of symptoms? The epidemiological literature clearly demonstrates that once a person has had an initial episode of low back pain, they are at increased risk of ongoing low back pain, of either the chronic or recurrent type. While it is commonly believed that acute back pain resolves spontaneously within two months in the majority of cases (Waddell, 1987), 35 to 60% of patients will still experience symptoms at three months (van den Hoogen et al, 1997; Von Korff & Saunders, 1996) while 10 to 25% will remain symptomatic at one year post-onset (van den Hoogen et al, 1997; Croft et al, 1998). In a large study conducted in an industrial setting, 62% of subjects experienced recurrence within the first year with 36% experiencing two or more recurrences (Bergquist-Ullman & Larsson, 1977).

recent prospective study, ongoing back pain was present in 71% of respondents at four year follow-up (Smith et al, 2004). Epidemiological statistics such as these suggest that, if the motor control changes observed in the presence of spinal dysfunction are intended to enhance spinal stability and thus control symptoms, they are not especially effective.

Further consideration of this controversy may be based upon an analysis of the clinical interventions which emerge from the adaptive and maladaptive interpretations. As developed initially by Richardson and colleagues, the motor re-education model of therapeutic exercise is based on the idea that the dysfunction noted in segmental muscles such as transversus abdominis and multifidus represents a form of maladaptive motor control error. As such they recommended a novel motor re-education approach (Richardson et al, 1999). This interpretation has received considerable support from the clinical community (Lee, 1999c; O'Sullivan, 2000; Jemmett, 2003) where it is appreciated that the rehabilitation of motor dysfunction necessitates an approach distinct from that utilized in the setting of muscle weakness. Undoubtedly, this knowledge is derived from the clinician's unique expertise with both orthopaedic and neurologic populations.

Alternatively, an adaptive interpretation, one which considers these motor control changes to be functional, might be expected to advocate for gross motor, anti-gravity exercises which improve the function of the multi-segmental muscles. Interestingly, this would likely result in a set of exercises similar to those in vogue when low back pain was believed to be associated with simple weakness of the trunk muscles. Although such exercises may be performed in a gentle fashion with little mechanical load developed across the lumbar spine (McGill, 2002b), they nonetheless represent a marked challenge to the neural control subsystem. In the authors' opinion, such exercises are likely to overwhelm, rather than rehabilitate, an already impaired neural control subsystem. From our clinical perspective, such interventions serve only to reinforce compensatory strategies, which, as described above, appear to be problematic in the long term.

An interesting feature of the adaptive vs. maladaptive controversy is that the argument appears to break down along professional lines. Those with physiotherapy backgrounds tend to favour the maladaptive interpretation (Richardson et al, 1999; Lee, 1999; O'Sullivan, 2000; Comerford & Mottram, 2001; Jemmett, 2003; Hodges & Moseley, 2003) while those with kinesiology or engineering backgrounds frequently argue for the adaptive interpretation (Cholewicki & McGill, 1996; Panjabi, 2003; van Dieen, 2003). Readers might wish to be aware of these divisions as they form their own opinions regarding this research. It is possible that professional or educational biases may influence both the reader's and the researcher's interpretations of this literature.

Ultimately, the motor control changes known to be present in patients with low back pain are both adaptive **and** maladaptive. Given the increased amplitudes of the NZ along with the anatomical and neuromuscular activation deficits seen in the setting of lumbar pathology, the neural control subsystem's increased activation of the multi-segmental muscles represents an effective and necessary strategy in the period immediately following the onset of symptoms. However, it would appear that the ongoing use of this strategy is neither efficient nor effective. This is likely due to the multi-segmental muscles being architecturally suited and neurophysiologically utilized for the purpose of regional, rather than segmental, motion generation and control. As such, therapeutic interventions designed to enhance these strategies may not result in optimal segmental motion control. Conversely, interventions which include exercises designed to restore the 'fine-tuning' function of muscles such as transversus abdominis and multifidus may be more likely to result in optimal segmental motion control and improved clinical outcomes. Indeed, a number of clinical outcomes studies have shown this motor re-education approach to have good efficacy in both acute and chronic populations with either low back or pelvic girdle pain (Hides et al, 1996; O'Sullivan et al, 1997; Hides et al, 2001; Brox et al, 2003; Niemisto et al, 2003; Shaughnessy & Caulfield, 2004).

Summary

The segmental spinal ROM is partitioned into the neutral zone (NZ) and the elastic zone (EZ). As described by Panjabi, functional spinal stability is concerned with optimal control of NZ motion and protection of the osseoligamentous tissues. This control and protection is provided by the active subsystem and coordinated by the neural control subsystem such that the amplitude of the NZ is maintained within tolerable limits. A variety of lumbar region muscles may function to control segmental spinal motion *via* the generation of intersegmental stiffness (figure 3.11a). Current architectural, biomechanical and neurophysiological evidence suggests that the most efficient are the deep segmental muscles of the trunk: the transversus abdominis, psoas, quadratus lumborum and the multifidus. The neural control subsystem utilizes both feedforward and feedback mechanisms to provide optimal activation of a number of muscles in meeting the simultaneous stability and mobility requirements of the lumbar spine.

With the onset of either traumatic or degenerative osseoligamentous pathology a marked loss of segmental stiffness develops. With experimentally induced trauma this correlates with a dramatic increase in the amplitude of the NZ. As measured in degenerative segments, the path of the instantaneous axis of rotation becomes larger and more chaotic. Concurrently, a number of neuromuscular deficits are present in patients with lumbar dysfunction (figure 3.11b). Generally, deep segmental muscles develop altered activation patterns along with a number of morphological and histochemical changes. In the presence of this dysfunction, the multi-segmental muscles are believed to be utilized by the neural control subsystem in an attempt to gain some measure of control over segmental motion. The increases in spinal load associated with this strategy along with the existence of ongoing symptoms in patients with either episodic or chronic histories suggests that this compensatory response is neither optimal nor especially satisfactory in the long term.

Every solution requires a problem.

Upon review of the current literature it is readily apparent that low back pain is a far more complex clinical problem than was suggested by more traditional models. It is certainly accepted that ligaments, vertebral endplates, intervertebral discs and z-joint capsules become pathologic. However, even when conclusively demonstrated using invasive and/or advanced imaging techniques (Laslett, 2004), diagnoses such as 'annular tear of the intervertebral disc' convey only a limited understanding of the patient's problem. Mere identification of the lesion type does not lead to a sufficient appreciation for the important sequelae which develop in association with such pathologies. Indeed, in light of the current literature, a continued emphasis on such a pathoanatomical approach is likely to divert our attention from more clinically important and identifiable features of the patient's presentation.

It is our opinion that the current research supports the hypothesis that a majority of patients with 'non-specific' or 'discogenic' low back pain present with a decrease in segmental stiffness (i.e., an increase in the amplitude of the NZ) along with altered motor control patterns affecting both the segmental and multi-segmental muscles. Further, it is proposed that a comprehensive and evidence-based manual therapy examination can provide the clinician with an appreciation for the nature and extent of these changes. Such a clinical appreciation will be sufficient to initiate an effective, patient-specific management plan - an effective solution based upon a more complete understanding of the underlying problem.

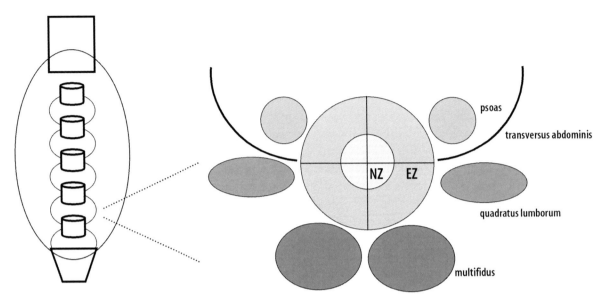

Figure 3.11a In the setting of a healthy spine, the neural control subsystem maintains spinal stability through a dynamic activation process whereby segmental and multisegmental muscles are utilized in a task-appropriate manner. Specifically, the segmental muscles are utilized to maintain normal neutral zone (NZ) amplitudes. The multi-segmental muscles are utilized to maintain regional postures and prevent buckling of the lumbar spine, a form of stability referred to as *Euler stability*.

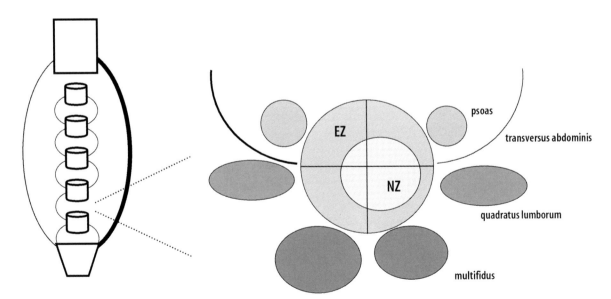

Figure 3.11b Schematic representation of a common pattern of changes in the lumbar spine associated with neuromusculoskeletal dysfunction. In the above example, osseoligamentous pathology has developed at the L4-5 level with symptoms experienced primarily on the right side. The segment's NZ is increased, there are morphological and motor control changes affecting the segmental muscles on the painful side, and activation of the multi-segmental muscles is increased. Although this increased activation of the multi-segmental muscles is likely a useful compensatory strategy limiting motion of the injured segment in the acute phase of healing, over time increased tissue loading, compromised respiratory function and a potential alteration of the segment's rotational axis suggest that this is a less than optimal long-term adaptation.

clinical reasoning & the segmental dysfunction model

THIS CHAPTER MARKS a transition from the scientific literature to the clinical reality and consists of two primary discussions. In the first, we consider the theoretical aspects of clinical reasoning through an examination of the retrospective and prospective models of clinical reasoning. In the second, we detail the segmental dysfunction model and describe four proposed sub-categories of segmental dysfunction which may be utilized to guide patient management. The chapter concludes with a hypothetical case study developed to highlight the clinical application of the segmental dysfunction model.

Clinical Reasoning in Orthopaedic Physiotherapy

IN THE PAST THIRTY YEARS the knowledge base and skill set within orthopaedic physiotherapy has grown substantially. Given this evolution, many jurisdictions have granted direct access privileges to licensed physiotherapists. As a result, many orthopaedic physiotherapists are now considered primary care clinicians and have far greater autonomy in terms of the assessment and management of their patients. As we begin the clinical section of this text it is important to discuss the construct of clinical reasoning. Clinical reasoning refers to the underlying cognitive processes fundamental to the diagnosis of pathology and the management of patients.

While all clinicians utilize clinical reasoning to guide their patient management decisions, there are significant and interesting differences between novices and experts regarding the manner and extent to which they use reasoning to form their clinical impressions (Jones, 1992; Custers et al, 2000). In general, novices tend to divide the clinical assessment into two discrete segments: an initial data gathering phase and an interpretive analytical phase. The novice considers these phases to be separate entities; in the first they are asking questions and performing tests. Once the data gathering is completed, the task of analyzing the data begins.

Experts on the other hand follow a classic scientific *hypothetico-deductive* process. This refers to a model of assessment whereby diagnostic hypotheses are formed, tested and confirmed in 'real-time'. The clinician develops, challenges and accepts or rejects a set of hypothetical diagnoses as a means of developing a differential diagnosis. The physical examination is used, in the majority of circumstances, to confirm or negate the differential diagnosis, rather than to elicit further data. The literature is consistent in its agreement that the prospective process typically employed by expert clinicians facilitates a more efficient assessment and yields a more accurate diagnosis (Jones, 1992; Terry & Higgs, 1993; Charlin et al, 2000).

Pattern Recognition

THE RECOGNITION OF CLINICAL patterns is fundamental to the hypothetico-deductive process (Jones, 1992; Custers et al., 2000). However, pattern recognition is by no means reserved for the domains of science and medicine. Indeed, all human learning is based on pattern recognition. The recognition of patterns allows us to be more efficient in virtually every aspect of our lives. Consider our awareness of the construct for 'automobile'. In order to appreciate a car as being a car, it is not necessary for us to fully identify and understand each car's component parts, their individual workings and their interactions with other component parts; we simply recognize the cognitive *pattern* developed at some point in our life for 'car'. The fact that one car has four doors, or another is bright yellow, or that another is full of rust and has no rear bumper does not distract us from our awareness that these are all 'cars'. We are able to attend to the primary salient features which lead to the recognition of 'car'.

Imagine what life would be like if we didn't interpret our world based on pattern recognition. Each time we saw a slightly different car, we would need to go through an extensive data analysis process, sorting through all the various similarities and variations, simply to arrive at the conclusion that - like the four door, blue sedan we saw a moment ago - this bright green hatchback with a red mountain bike attached to a roof-rack is also a 'car'. However, inefficiency is not the only negative outcome associated with an avoidance of pattern

recognition. Of even greater concern is the risk of becoming so caught up in their irrelevant differences that we fail to recognize them both as 'cars'.

The act of reading provides another example of pattern recognition. How efficient would reading be if each word had to be analyzed letter by letter, sounded out as early readers do? Such a process could even detract from the reader's ability to grasp the fundamentals of the story. The majority of people over the age of seven have learned to recognize the visual pattern of a word rather than engaging in the painstaking exercise of sorting through the various combinations of letters one by one. Indeed, as people become even more expert at reading, pattern recognition is extended beyond individual words to whole phrases. We learn by experience to expect certain words to follow others simply by having been exposed to that pattern over and over again.

To illustrate the concept of pattern recognition differences between experts and novices, Mark Jones offered the example of two chess players, one a master and the other a novice (Jones, 1992). When the novice looks at the pieces in play on a chess board, they can only identify the individual pieces. The expert not only identifies the pieces, they appreciate their *meaning* or significance; they are able to 'see' potential strategic patterns of attack and defense. If the expert and novice are asked to quickly view *randomly* placed pieces on a chess board, they will perform relatively equally in terms of their ability to reproduce the position of the pieces. However, if the pieces are placed on the board as per a true strategic pattern, the expert reproduces the pieces more quickly and accurately than the novice. The master chess player quickly recognizes the pattern and thus has no need to recall all the individual pieces and their positions. Unable to see the pattern, the novice must attempt to interpret thirty-two separate and apparently unrelated pieces of information. The expert is able to 'see' patterns in part because they have learned that not all pieces on the board are of equal significance in all strategic circumstances. Certain combinations of certain chess pieces are more powerful than others. It is the relative relationships between such pieces that form the patterns recognized by the master player.

In medicine, a variety of common examples illustrate the concept of pattern recognition as being an important component of the diagnostic process. When a physician encounters a patient with a fever accompanied by progressive, non-traumatic lower right abdominal pain, a clinical pattern suggestive of acute appendicitis readily comes to mind. Likewise when a middle aged patient complains of fatigue, weight gain and increased urinary frequency, their symptomatic pattern is recognized as being strongly suggestive of type II diabetes. In either of these scenarios, the patient may well have other complaints in addition to those listed. A critical feature of expert clinical pattern recognition is the ability to attend to the significant items which comprise a certain diagnostic pattern while appreciating other complaints as being either secondary or even insignificant in the context of that specific presentation. In both cases, rather than ordering a plethora of tests, the expert clinician need only order the one or two tests necessary to confirm their suspected diagnosis.

If people did not comprehend the world through a process based upon pattern recognition, we could not begin to function given the enormous barrage of data that we must interpret on a continuous basis. Interestingly, student and novice health care professionals, in general, tend not to employ pattern recognition when faced with the significant amount of data that develops each time they encounter a new patient. This is an understandable phenomena considering the limited knowledge and clinical experience that novices possess relative to experts. Given the potential consequences of being incorrect when diagnosing a new patient, it is not surprising that novices are reluctant to forego a massive data gathering process and trust in their ability to recognize clinical patterns. Indeed, in clinical practice as in chess, it is the ability to quickly and accurately recognize patterns which distinguishes the expert from the novice.

Retrospective & Prospective Clinical Reasoning

To this point clinical reasoning has been discussed in terms of the novice and the expert approach. This is a fair representation of the literature which has been developed primarily in the medical education field, where clinical reasoning is often considered in terms of the novice and expert physician. However, while there are significant differences in terms of clinical reasoning skills between novice and expert physicians, there are also significant differences between health care professions in terms of the clinical reasoning models promoted by their respective academic communities. As such, from this point forward, rather than discussing clinical reasoning in terms of novice and expert performance, we will review two forms of clinical reasoning, retrospective and prospective.

The Retrospective Model of Clinical Reasoning

The retrospective clinical reasoning model is summarized in figure 4.1. The retrospective model divides the assessment into two discrete phases: a 'data gathering' phase and a 'data analysis' phase. In conducting the assessment of a new patient, the retrospective model requires the clinician to ask many questions and perform a multitude of tests. The clinician often performs a more or less standardized battery of regional tests based on the idea that it is necessary to perform a 'complete examination'. The clinician's skill at such tasks may indeed be excellent. Yet, by the completion of the data gathering phase, the clinician has amassed only a lengthy list of apparently discrete findings, each assumed to be of equal diagnostic significance or value.

Typically, neither the relative importance of each finding, nor the relationships between findings will have been established using a retrospective approach. With equal significance assigned to each test result, the clinician then

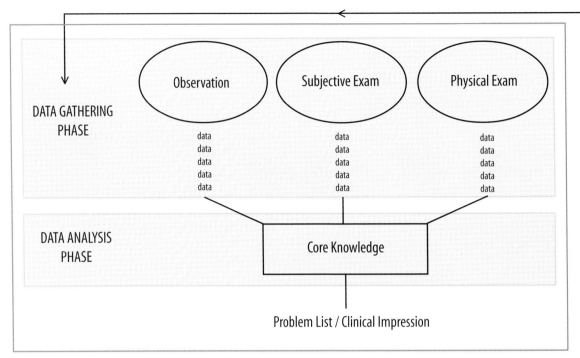

Figure 4.1 The retrospective model of clinical reasoning. The examination is divided into a data gathering phase and a data analysis phase.

reviews a large amount of data, attempting to identify relationships or patterns leading to a clinical impression. The reasoning process is employed only after the data is compiled; as such, reasoning has little opportunity to influence the assessment process as it unfolds. As a result, the clinician's ability to recognize the emergence of a clinical pattern is greatly limited. A key risk associated with this form of reasoning is the tendency for the clinician to see a variety of independent problems rather than a clinical pattern. Related to the retrospective model of clinical reasoning is the problem solving approach to patient management. As individual findings become identified as clinical problems, treatment comes to emphasize the resolution of these 'discrete' problems rather than attempting to manage the underlying pathology.

The Prospective Model of Clinical Reasoning

THE PROSPECTIVE MODEL of clinical reasoning is presented in figure 4.2. Unlike the retrospective model, there is no temporal or procedural separation of the assessment, reasoning and analytical processes. Reasoning, hypothesis development and the building of a differential diagnosis are inter-related, with each influencing the overall process as it develops. The assessment, rather than being highly structured in terms of content and sequencing, is more improvisational. However, this should not be interpreted as haphazard. Improvisational jazz musicians are highly skilled in terms of technique yet even more so in their ability to recognize what is required of them within the current performance. Likewise, prospective clinical reasoning requires the clinician to be capable of recognizing the emergence of clinical patterns, generating clinical hypotheses

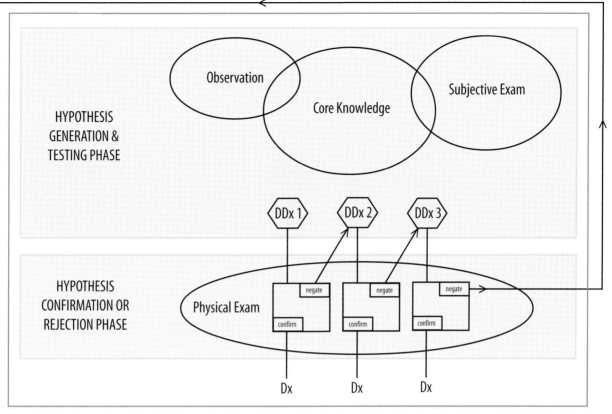

Figure 4.2 The prospective model of clinical reasoning. The subjective examination is used to develop the differential diagnosis (DDx). The physical examination consists of a patient-specific set of tests selected to confirm the most likely diagnosis (DDx1) while negating competing diagnoses (DDx2 and DDx3). If none of the possible diagnoses are confirmed on physical examination, the clinician may need to conduct a retrospective examination.

based on these patterns and then responding appropriately in terms of hypothesis testing. Under a prospective reasoning paradigm, the subjective examination is utilized to develop the differential diagnosis and the physical examination to confirm the differential diagnosis. A patient and context-specific set of physical examination items is selected in order to both confirm the suspected diagnosis and negate potential alternate diagnoses. The physical examination is not used as a data collection instrument as it is under the retrospective model. Each patient's unique presentation influences the content and structure of the assessment. The clinician begins to generate a list of hypothetical diagnoses as soon as they observe the patient entering the examination room. During the course of the subjective examination, as a possible diagnosis is generated, the next question is used specifically to test this hypothesis. The patient's

response will either support or negate the potential diagnosis. If the patient's response supports the hypothesis, the following question is chosen specifically to further challenge the same hypothesis. If the answer negates the hypothetical diagnosis, the clinician may or may not change course, depending on the relative strength of that specific item.

Both the subjective and objective examinations evolve along a curve unique to each patient as the clinician tests the credibility of their hypothesis, or differential diagnosis. If each successive piece of subjective data strengthens the working hypothesis, they continue along that diagnostic path; if they find good evidence to abandon a certain hypothesis they begin the process anew with the next most likely diagnosis. Once a reasonable differential diagnosis is established, the clinician selects a set of objective tests chosen for their ability to confirm the most likely diagnosis and negate other potential diagnoses. When a series of subjective and objective items has both confirmed the most likely diagnosis and refuted other potential diagnoses, the clinician concludes their examination.

While it may be unavoidable that students utilize the retrospective model until they have gained sufficient experience to apply a more prospective model, they should be made aware of the advantages and disadvantages of these two approaches. Likewise, even experienced clinicians who have been professionally socialized towards the retrospective model will benefit from an awareness of the prospective model and its efficacy. As stated above, the prospective model consistently results in more efficient and accurate diagnoses, largely due to its facilitation of clinical pattern recognition (Elstein et al, 1978; Jones, 1992; Custers et al, 2000).

Potential Pitfalls Associated with Prospective Clinical Reasoning

ALTHOUGH IT IS ACCEPTED that prospective clinical reasoning (e.g., pattern recognition and the hypothetico-deductive process) results in more effective and efficient patient management, potential problems in the execution of this approach have been described (Jones, 1992; Custers et al, 2000). Generally these are related to a novice's relative lack of knowledge and experience, or to an experienced clinician failing to either challenge a diagnostic hypothesis sufficiently or fully consider all diagnostic possibilities.

A limited ability to develop a reasonable differential diagnosis

This may be relatively difficult to modify as it is strongly related to experience. However, students and clinicians can be expected to improve their ability to develop a differential diagnosis if they are encouraged and supported in their early attempts to consider, and look for, relationships between subjective findings and causal mechanisms (i.e., clinical patterns). In the authors' opinion, an important barrier to this evolution, perhaps specific to orthopaedic physiotherapy, is a tendency to overvalue the clinician's physical examination skill set. While more advanced examination and treatment skills are without question an important part of professional development, all clinicians, regardless of the extent of their current 'manual therapy' skill set will see their success with patient management increase substantially with the application of a more prospective clinical reasoning model. If the adoption of prospective clinical reasoning is stunted by an overemphasis on skill set development, the clinician's capacity to optimally manage their patients will be unnecessarily limited.

Confirmation Bias

It is not uncommon for clinicians to have a set of preferred diagnostic hypotheses. Therefore, they must guard against any tendency to overemphasize findings which support a favorite diagnosis or pay inadequate attention to those findings which negate it. Custers and colleagues stated "in our view, the confirmation bias is a natural risk of the hypothetico-deductive process" (Custers, 2000). The clinician must perform adequate due diligence with each and every patient.

Premature Closure

Related to the confirmation bias is the error of accepting a hypothesis too early in the process without fully exploring other possibilities. This can occur when the clinician moves too quickly into the hypothesis confirmation phase of the assessment. Sufficient attention must be given to fully exploring all possibilities during the hypothesis generation and testing phase. The authors suggest that all efforts should be made to develop at least three items for the differential diagnosis and then rigorously explore them *via* an appropriate set of physical examination items.

Excessive Data Gathering

The primary concern with excessive data gathering is that it represents an unreasoned approach to clinical practice and generates a potentially confusing volume of data (Terry & Higgs, 1993) which might lead the clinician away from an understanding of the underlying problem. While excessive data collection has been described as being a feature of the retrospective clinical model, it may also occur in the prospective model. Clinicians must perform a thorough assessment without becoming excessive in their use of physical examination items. If the clinician applies a patient-specific battery of tests sufficient to fully confirm the differential diagnosis and negate competing hypotheses, they will have conducted a thorough yet non-excessive assessment.

Errors in Logic and Reasoning

Clinicians must use caution when making inferences about causality; this is especially problematic when utilizing a pathoanatomical model. For example, if a patient has significant nerve root compromise they will likely have 'positive' findings on neurodynamic testing. However, it is an error in reasoning to assume that if a patient has 'positive' neurodynamic findings they will have significant nerve root compromise.

Retrospective & Prospective Reasoning in Low Back Pain

THE CONCEPT OF PATTERN recognition has been described as being a key component of prospective clinical reasoning and expert clinical practice. While it is true that experience is a necessary element in pattern recognition, even more fundamental is a knowledge of the underlying construct. If a child were never taught the basic concept for 'car', they might go on for many years believing that blue sedans were fundamentally different from red convertibles. Similarly in clinical practice, if the underlying pathophysiology of a disorder is not known, it is virtually impossible to recognize any true relatedness amongst a certain set of symptoms. It is the identification of the fundamental pathology underlying the disorder which allows clinicians to assign appropriate levels of significance to a variety of symptoms such that a predictable, consistent and clinically useful pattern may emerge, one which leads to a superior model of management.

For example, the pathology underlying type II diabetes – impaired insulin regulation - is well established. With this understanding of the inherent pathophysiology, it becomes possible to recognize the symptomatic pattern of fatigue, obesity and increased urinary frequency as being pathognomonic for the disease. Other symptoms which might exist concurrently may be recognized as being either secondary or unrelated. For instance, *difficulty concentrating* as being secondary to fatigue and poorly controlled blood glucose levels and *heart burn* as being unrelated altogether.

If the underlying pathophysiology of type II diabetes were not understood, clinical management might take one of two paths. *Via* the first, clinicians might treat each symptom as a discrete entity, as per a problem solving model, with each complaint being considered an independent malady in need of its own 'management'. Alternatively, individual clinicians or groups of clinicians might develop symptom classification schemes based primarily upon clinical expertise and opinion. With either approach, any clinical patterns which do emerge will have been developed at least somewhat arbitrarily rather than through an evidence-based understanding of the cause and effect relationships between the underlying pathology and the patient's symptoms. Orthopaedic clinicians will likely recognize the similarities between this hypothetical example and the current reality regarding our management of patients with low back pain. Without an understanding of the pathomechanics of low back pain, not only are we prevented from recognizing meaningful clinical patterns, we remain mired in that situation described by the classic axiom – **where the diagnosis is vague, the treatments are many.**

The problem of low back pain typifies the challenges inherent in managing a condition in which the underlying pathology is poorly understood. It has been recognized for some time that the underlying pathomechanics of low back pain were largely unknown (Nachemson, 1985; Riihimaki, 1991). As described in chapter one, the management of patients with low back pain using a pathoanatomical model has been relatively unimpressive with no single approach showing marked superiority over another (Hurley et al, 2004). Given the inability to identify the cause or source of the patient's symptoms it has been difficult to apply prospective clinical reasoning to the problem of low back pain in an effective fashion. We have been limited either to gross categorizations such as discogenic or 'non-specific' low back pain, or to largely unproven, anecdotally driven diagnostic schemes which vary from one expert to another. Neither has been especially helpful in the development of predictable and effective patient management strategies. Thus, if clinical outcomes are to improve, it is imperative that an evidence-based definition of the pathomechanics of low back pain be established.

The pathomechanics of lumbar pathology can be anticipated to be complex and multi-factorial. Eventually, it is likely that both proximate and ultimate factors will have been identified. Ultimate factors will probably be found through molecular and genetic studies and will eventually explain, for example, why the human intervertebral disc experiences a degenerative process over the lifespan. However, their conclusive identification and any resultant therapeutic or preventive interventions remain some years away. Proximate factors are those which are more directly related to the immediate onset of pathology. Given the literature as reviewed in chapters two and three, we propose that there is sufficient evidence to define a consistent set of proximate pathomechanical factors, consistently seen in a majority of patients with lumbar pathology. These proximate factors, detailed in the following section, constitute the basis for an evidence-based clinical pattern, one which may be objectively appreciated on clinical examination.

However, an appreciation of this definition requires that we 'let go' of a variety of traditional beliefs about the spine and the nature of low back pain. Not the least of these beliefs involves the validity of the pathoanatomical model itself (Varamini & Jam, 2005a). As stated by Panjabi, "… in a real-life situation an individual spinal component is seldom injured alone … several anatomical components of the spinal column are injured, but to varying degrees" (Panjabi, 2003). Thus, low back pain is rarely the result of pathology affecting a single spinal structure or tissue, nor is it possible, on clinical examination, or even with modern imaging techniques, to develop a comprehensive and accurate pathoanatomical diagnosis in most instances of lumbar pathology.

The Segmental Dysfunction Model of Lumbar Pathology

THIS SECTION BEGINS WITH an examination of the proposed pathomechanics and etiology of lumbar pathology as per the segmental dysfunction model (SDM) and as supported by the current literature (note that a comprehensive review of this research is found in chapter three). A discussion of the manner in which this underlying dysfunction may manifest symptomatically is followed by a description of the model's application in clinical practice. Finally, we present a categorization scheme consisting of four segmental dysfunction subgroups developed to assist clinicians in their clinical decision making.

Pathomechanics of Lumbar Pathology

THE LITERATURE IS CONSISTENT in its identification of two critical deficits which are present in a majority of patients with lumbar dysfunction: altered segmental stiffness and a loss of normal motor control affecting the segmental and multi-segmental muscles. Indeed, there is evidence that not only do these deficits tend to co-exist in patients with low back pain but that they may in fact be related in a cause and effect fashion (McGill, 2003; Solomonow, 1998). Together, this pattern of segmental dysfunction has also been described as a clinical instability (Panjabi, 1992).

This interdependent set of deficits develops regardless of whether the underlying lesion involves the intervertebral disc, the vertebral endplate, a spinal ligament, a zygapophysial joint tissue or the vertebrae itself. It should be noted that the SDM allows for the traditional pathoanatomical view that specific spinal tissues become pathological in patients with low back pain. However, the SDM argues that lumbar dysfunction typically involves pathology affecting more than a single osseoligamentous structure and that it is not possible, in a majority of cases, to accurately

identify those injured structures *via* the clinical examination. As such, the SDM is not concerned with identifying *the* pathological structure. Instead, the emphasis is on identifying the location of the symptom generating motion segment(s) and developing a clinical appreciation for the extent and nature of the articular stiffness and neuro-muscular changes impacting that segment(s).

Altered Segmental Stiffness

Both *in vivo* and *in vitro* studies have identified significant changes in segmental stiffness as being a consistent finding in the presence of lumbar pathology. *In vitro* studies of the load tolerating capacity of the lumbar spine (Oxland & Panjabi, 1992) along with estimates of segmental stiffness as predicted *via* biomechanical models (Cholewicki & McGill, 1996) both demonstrate a dramatic loss of segmental stiffness at the onset of osseoligamentous pathology. Indeed, it has been stated that a marked increase in NZ amplitude (as develops with an abrupt loss of segmental stiffness) is the most powerful indicator of the presence of osseoligamentous pathology (Panjabi, 1992). Gertzbein's studies of segmental motion quality in the presence of mild to moderate degenerative pathology (Gertzbein et al, 1985 & 1986) are suggestive of similar changes in the presence of non-traumatic pathologies. Thus, findings of this type support the statement that lumbar pathology necessarily involves an alteration in the pathological segment's stiffness characteristics.

In most clinical presentations a decrease in osscoligamentous stiffness (synonymous with an increase in segmental compliance) at the dysfunctional segment is anticipated (Oxland & Panjabi, 1992; Panjabi, 2003). This will be readily apparent upon examination of the passive subsytem *via* typical 'manual therapy' examination. Interestingly, in some situations, this loss of osseoligamentous stiffness will be so overlaid with excessive activity of the multi-segmental muscles that the motion segment is compressed (Lee, 1999d). A result of this compensatory but excessive multi-segmental activity may be a shift of the segment's axis of rotation, resulting in a dynamically hypomobile segment. Where severe degenerative changes have developed, an increase in segmental stiffness (or a decrease in compliance) may be expected (Panjabi, 1992b; Gertzbein et al, 1986).

Altered Motor Control

It is critical to recall that the healthy human spinal column is in fact an inherently unstable structure with a critical load of no more than 90N (Crisco et al, 1992; Panjabi et al, 1998). In the lumbar spine, a wide range of osseoligamentous pathology will develop with physiological loads of between 20 and 90N (Oxland & Panjabi, 1992). This is far below published estimates of the spinal loads associated with activities of daily living, as well as occupational and sports activities in which spinal load can exceed several thousand newtons (Cholewicki et al., 1991). Thus, the neurological and muscular systems are critical to the maintenance of spinal stability (Panjabi, 1992a).

The characteristic motor control changes present in patients with lumbar dysfunction involve impaired control of the deep segmental muscles coupled with a compensatory activation of the multi-segmental muscles (Hodges, 2004). Evidence of deep muscle impairment has been reported *via* histological, anatomical and neuro-physiological investigations (Rantanen et al, 1993; Hides et al, 1994; Hodges & Richardson, 1996; Zhao et al, 2000; Barker et al, 2004; MacDonald et al, 2004). The transversus abdominis muscle becomes delayed in its activation as do the deep fibers of the multifidus muscle. In addition, losses in cross sectional area or muscle volume have been reported in both the multifidus and psoas muscles adjacent to the dysfunctional lumbar segment (Hides et al, 1994; Barker et al, 2004). There is good evidence that these and/or other such deficits persist despite the resolution of symptoms in acute low back pain (Hides et al, 1996) and for at least five years following spinal surgery (Rantanen et al, 1993). Evidence of excessive activation in multi-segmental muscles such as the erector spinae has been reported (Ferguson et al, 2004; Silfies et al, *in*

press) and is commonly observed in clinical practice in the form of increased paraspinal muscle 'tone'.

Etiology of Lumbar Pathology

THE SDM considers typical* neuromusculoskeletal lumbar pathology to develop *via* one of two routes – degenerative changes or trauma. Degenerative disc disease and osteoarthritis are well described in the lumbar spine as are both central and lateral recess stenosis. However, our concept of trauma requires some degree of modification from the traditional. Trauma involving the structures of the spinal column may occur as a result of a single event, or a series of events, where the loads transmitted to the passive subsystem eventually exceed its failure point (Oxland & Panjabi, 1992; Panjabi et al, 1998). Such injury will lead to the pattern of dysfunction affecting the passive, active and neural control subsystems described previously in chapter three. Thus, while trauma may involve the significant loads seen in automobile collisions, falls and impact sports such as football, rugby or hockey, more benign events may nonetheless result in traumatic loading of the osseoligamentous spine should the neuromuscular systems fail to adequately protect vulnerable spinal tissues (Panjabi, 1992a; Preuss & Fung, 2005). Indeed, the SDM's ability to predict or account for such common injury mechanisms is one of its key strengths.

Trauma secondary to a benign event may occur purely as a result of neuromuscular error or as the eventual sequelae of repeated micro-trauma or creep affecting the osseoligamentous tissues. Given the low failure point of the osseoligamentous lumbar spine, it is plausible that injury of the passive subsystem could occur as a result of a relatively benign event (bending, reaching, even simply walking) if the neural control subsystem failed to either correctly anticipate the stability requirements of a given segment or adequately recruit a specific component of the active subsystem at the appropriate time (Panjabi, 1992a). This intriguing hypothesis was provided some experimental support by Cholewicki and McGill

---

*Typical refers to neuromusculoskeletal (orthopaedic) pathology and is thus exclusive of systemic disease, infection, or neoplasm.

who reported the capture of such an event while conducting an experiment with trained powerlifters (Cholewicki & McGill, 1992). Alternatively, Solomonow and colleagues have demonstrated the potential for osseoligamentous creep to lead to segmental laxity, *via* decreased tensioning in the spinal ligaments with a resultant loss of reflexive activation of the lumbar paraspinal muscles (Solomonow et al, 1998; Olson et al, 2004).

Symptom Manifestation

GIVEN THE TRI-PLANAR nature of lumbar segmental biomechanics, the pathomechanics as outlined above and the potential for both mechanical and chemical irritants to affect any combination of osseoligamentous, muscular and/or neurologic tissues adjacent to the dysfunctional segment(s), a wide variety of symptomatic presentations must be allowed for under the SDM. It is feasible that patients may present with low back pain (unilateral or bilateral), lower extremity symptoms or a combination of both. A patient might report unilateral low back pain along with contralateral lower extremity symptoms. Alternatively, a patient lacking a reasonable history for peripheral pathology but who has a history of either episodic or chronic low back pain, may well have a segmental dysfunction mechanism responsible for their purely peripheral symptoms. In some situations, true peripheral pathology may arise as a result of a given patient's unique compensatory pattern of activation of the multi-segmental muscles. A thorough history, conducted in a prospective fashion and underpinned with an appreciation for the SDM, will result in a reasonable differential diagnosis in the majority of circumstances.

Clinical Application

THE FUNDAMENTAL KNOWLEDGE base and skill set of orthopaedic physiotherapy has traditionally involved the assessment and treatment of articular

and muscular dysfunction. There is excellent existing correspondence between the SDM and modern manual therapy practice. A detailed description of physiotherapeutic assessment and management as per the SDM is presented in chapters five and six. By way of an overview, the practical application of the SDM may described as follows:

Identify the Symptom Generating Segment

A variety of subjective and objective findings will provide clinical evidence* as to the location of the primary symptom generating segment. For example, a radicular pattern of pain into the anterior aspect of the thigh is suggestive of L3-4 segmental dysfunction. Confirming tests would include careful observation of the lumbar spine during active movements, segmental compliance testing, segmental integrity testing and palpation for multifidus muscle volume (such tests are described in chapter five). An increase in segmental compliance noted on articular testing along with a loss of multifidus volume at L3-4 would confirm the differential diagnosis of an L3-4 segmental dysfunction or clinical instability. The ability of the manual therapy examination to identify the symptom generating segment in the lumbar spine has been investigated (Hides et al, 1994). In this study, manual therapy findings indicating the level of the symptom generating segment were correlated with the level at which a unilateral loss of multifidus CSA was found *via* ultrasound imaging in 24 of 26 subjects.

Assess the Stiffness or Compliance Characteristics of the Lumbar Spine

Traditional manual therapy techniques of articular examination are utilized within the SDM to provide the clinician with an appreciation for the segmental stiffness or compliance characteristics of the lumbar region. The techniques themselves are not novel; however, the clinician's interpretation of the data obtained through the application of these techniques must be modified to remain in

*Clinical evidence must include both confirming and negating findings from each of the subjective and objective examinations.

keeping with existing evidence. While some of these tests are traditionally described as segmental *motion* tests, recent evidence negates the idea that segmental motion can be appreciated *via* a manual therapy examination. For example, radiographic and functional MRI studies of segmental motion during a posterior to anterior (PA) mobilization in the lumbar and cervical spine have shown that the expected anterior translation of one vertebrae relative to its segmental partner does not occur; instead, the spine simply bows into an extension-like curve (Lee & Evans, 1997; Powers et al, 2003; Kulig et al, 2004; Lee et al, 2005).

However, other manual therapy tests – such as the *passive accessory intervertebral motion test* – are intended to provide the clinician with an understanding of the status of the passive tissues at the segment's end range of motion. As such, these tests do not provide data regarding segmental motion but of segmental stiffness or compliance at the outer limit of the elastic zone. Historically, techniques of this type have been described as tests of the joint's 'end feel' (Cyriax, 1982). We propose that such tests are useful in developing a clinical appreciation for the stiffness/compliance status throughout the lumbar spine and, as such, may be used effectively as part of a comprehensive manual therapy examination. These tests along with their application and interpretation are described in detail in chapter five.

Assess the Status of the Segmental and Multi-Segmental Muscles of the Lumbar Spine

The manual therapy clinician may develop a clinical appreciation for the performance of the segmental and multi-segmental muscles of the lumbar spine *via* careful observation and palpation as well as through the use of ultrasound imaging. Given the clinical significance of the motor impairments affecting the deep segmental muscles, special attention is given to the status of the transversus abdominis and multifidus muscles as well as multi-segmental muscles such the diaphragm, rectus abdominis, external oblique and erector spinae. Again, these tests are described in detail in chapter five.

Assess the Patient's Self-Perception of Disability

As discussed in chapter one, each patient's psychosocial status will impact on their ability to achieve a successful rehabilitation outcome. While it remains controversial as to whether psychological or cognitive issues are most significant in this regard, it is recognized that a wide spectrum of psychosocial factors influence the development of disability (Pincus et al., 2002b). In our experience, the extent to which the patient's reported degree of disability correlates with the clinician's impression of the patient's condition is an important prognostic indicator or predictor of rehabilitative success. When a good 'fit' exists between clinician and patient in terms of their interpretation of the patient's condition, rehabilitative outcomes seem to be related primarily to the severity of the patient's physical status or segmental dysfunction and are thus highly predictable. However, when there is poor correlation, as in the situation where the clinician appreciates only a mild degree of physical pathology yet the patient reports a high degree of disability, rehabilitative outcomes tend to be poor with protracted durations of treatment, higher costs and typically little change in the patient's functional status. Thus, it is important that the clinician assess for the patient's perceptions regarding the extent of their disability using valid and reliable screening tools. The Roland-Morris Disability Questionnaire and the Oswestry Disability Questionnaire are each described as valid, reliable tools which may be utilized to efficiently assess a patient's self-concept of disability specific to their lower back symptoms (Roland & Fairbank, 2000).

Provide Appropriate Management

As in virtually all clinical situations, patient management decisions under the SDM are based upon examination findings. Using a prospective reasoning approach the clinician examines the patient, arrives at a diagnosis and prognosis and takes appropriate action based upon their impression of the patient's condition. Depending on the specific circumstances of a given patient's case, this will typically involve treatment of the patient's underlying articular and neuromuscular dysfunction. While we have proposed that the pathomechanics of lumbar pathology include altered segmental stiffness and impaired motor control, each patient will present with a relatively unique pattern of segmental dysfunction (clinical instability) resulting in a wide range of potential clinical presentations. Sources of variation include the number of dysfunctional segmental levels, whether the patient's dysfunction involves a uni-directional or multi-directional instability, the extent and nature of their motor control impairments and whether or not there is evidence of nerve root compromise. An overview consisting of twelve patterns of segmental dysfunction, their characteristic findings on examination, their prognosis and appropriate management is presented in chapter six.

It must be remembered that appropriate management may involve the decision not to treat a given patient. If the clinician appreciates the patient's segmental dysfunction to be sufficiently severe, optimal management might involve referral to the patient's family physician with a recommendation for orthopaedic or neurosurgical consultation. Alternatively, in any clinical circumstance where there is little or no objective evidence of segmental dysfunction, the physiotherapy clinician is obligated by the constructs of ethical practice to recognize the patient's condition as being outside their scope of practice and to refer on to a more appropriate clinician. In our opinion this is most critical in the situation where there is poor correlation between the clinician's findings and the patient's level of disability and specifically when the clinician can find little evidence of segmental dysfunction yet the patient describes a high level of symptom-related disability. Such patients certainly require intervention. However, appropriate management in these situations must be recognized as existing outside the skill set and knowledge base of most orthopaedic physiotherapists. In identifying a lack of objective

evidence supportive of a problem likely to be amenable to physiotherapeutic intervention, the clinician has indeed provided the patient, and the greater health care system, with a valuable professional service.

General Categories of Segmental Dysfunction

IN RECENT YEARS, the identification of a clinically meaningful classification system for patients with 'non-specific' low back pain has been the focus of much literature (Borkan et al, 1998; Fritz, 1998; Koes, 2004; Mannion, 2004; van Tulder, 2004; Varamini & Jam, 2005b). It has been argued that if current management and prevention strategies are to be improved, the identification of patient subgroups is critical (Bouter et al, 2003).

The segmental dysfunction model of lumbar pathology is based on the concept that each of the active, passive and neural control subsystems functions normally or adequately in the absence of lumbar spine pathology and that, to some extent, each subsystem functions abnormally in the presence of pathology. Clinically, such dysfunction occurs in clusters, or patterns, rather than in single isolated subsystems. In fact, patients consistently present with some degree of dysfunction in each.

As discussed previously, most patients with lumbar dysfunction present with an impairment of the segmental stabilizing and multi-segmental postural muscles along with alterations in segmental stiffness. These findings may be present at a variety of segments and in various combinations including the symptom generating segment alone or both the symptom generating segment and some adjacent lumbar segment, the sacroiliac joint or the hip joint. The fact that we can now identify a consistent set of pathomechanical features present in most patients allows for the development of a clinically relevant classification system which may be expected to positively impact on the management of our patients.

Table 4.1 presents an overview of the four fundamental categories of segmental dysfunction, or clinical instability, encountered in lumbar spine populations. These four general categories are expandable to account for the wide variety of possible combinations of other patient-specific features including the presence or absence of nerve root compromise, uni-directional or a multi-directional instabilities and either uni-level or multi-level segmental dysfunction. A description of twelve such clinical patterns along with their prognosis and suggested management is presented in chapter six.

Table 4.1 Categories of Segmental Dysfunction

Category	Passive Subsystem	Active Subsystem
Type 1 Clinical Instability	decreased segmental stiffness at symptom generating segment	impaired segmental muscle function
Type 2 Clinical Instability	decreased segmental stiffness at symptom generating segment	impaired segmental muscle function with excessive multi-segmental muscle co-contraction
Type 3 Clinical Instability	decreased segmental stiffness at symptom generating segment perpetuated by increased stiffness at an adjacent segment	impaired segmental muscle function with or without excessive multi-segmental muscle co-contraction
Type 4 Clinical Instability	increased segmental stiffness at symptom generating segment	impaired segmental muscle function with or without excessive multi-segmental muscle co-contraction

The Segmental Dysfunction Model Applied:
A Case Study Comparing Prospective Reasoning & Problem Solving in Neuromusculoskeletal Physiotherapy

PROSPECTIVE CLINICAL REASONING in general and the SDM in particular allows for the fact that the same finding (e.g., radiating lower limb pain) can have varying degrees of significance depending on the clinical context in which it occurs. This assignment of context-dependent importance aids in 'real-time' hypothesis building and reduces the risk of the clinician considering each finding to be a discrete problem requiring its own treatment (Custers et al., 2000). For example, consider a patient with chronic low back pain ('discrete' problem 1), who experiences increased back pain along with radiating lower extremity pain ('discrete' problem 2) if she sits for longer than 20 minutes ('discrete' problem 3). Treatment based upon a traditional model of lumbar pathology and retrospective clinical reasoning might include pain modalities for the lumbar spine and lower extremity along with 'functional' rehabilitation in which the patient is conditioned to tolerate longer periods of sitting. From the perspective of an integrated prospective clinical reasoning and segmental dysfunction model, the patient's symptoms would be appreciated as being secondary to a lumbar segmental dysfunction. The patient's articular, neuromuscular and neurodynamic status would be ascertained and managed. The patient's symptoms would be monitored and expected to improve as the primary deficit – their segmental dysfunction – improved.

The phrase 'problem solving model' may have different meanings for different people. Problem solving is only one of the processes utilized in clinical reasoning. To illustrate, consider three different clinicians each attempting to manage the same female patient who presents with a five month history of insidious onset lower quadrant symptoms. She has been referred to physical therapy by her family physician with the diagnosis of 'hip tendonitis/iliotibial band syndrome'.

The first clinician approaches this clinical situation as a matter of problem list management. This 'problem solving' clinician identifies that the patient cannot fully adduct her hip, that she has weakness in her external rotators and hip abductors and that she has pain throughout the L4 dermatome. There is tenderness along the lateral aspect of the thigh and posterior buttock. The clinician then attempts to treat this patient by correcting these various, and apparently discrete, problems.

The second clinician identifies the same list of deficits as well as the fact that the patient has a moderate degree of clinical instability at the L3-4 motion segment. Recognizing the primary physical dysfunction in this case to be the segmental dysfunction, they plan to treat the L3-4 segment. This clinician has recognized the clinical pattern and is therefore significantly closer to a comprehensive appreciation for this patient's presentation. However, they have not taken all relevant factors into account.

The third clinician, who happens to be a male, identifies *via* the history the same clinical pattern of lumbar segmental dysfunction and further suspects, based on his observation of the patient's gait, that she is likely hypomobile through her hips. However, he notes also that the patient has had similar symptoms sporadically for six years and is currently being managed by her family physician for depression (the patient will state only that this is secondary to having been physically assaulted by an unknown male assailant seven months previously). This clinician reasons that, while the patient's symptoms are likely due to an L3-4 clinical instability, possibly perpetuated by a lack of extension in her hips, her current psychosocial status may not be compatible with assessment or treatment by a male clinician.

This clinician has identified not only a more complete clinical pattern of physical dysfunction, but has also taken into account the patient's psychosocial status. In this case, while appropriate physical management of the patient would involve treatment of the L3-4 segmental dysfunction, the clinician recognizes that his clinical efforts are very likely to be incompatible with the patient's current psychosocial status. As such, the clinician might decide to advocate on the patient's behalf for more comprehensive psychological management and to forego physiotherapeutic treatment until such time as the patient would be more at ease with physical handling. Alternatively, he may decide to refer the patient to a female clinician, in the hope that this might lessen the patient's anxiety with regard to physical handling, and permit a more efficient resolution of the patient's segmental dysfunction.

Despite the range of clinical impressions developed by these three hypothetical clinicians, the problem solving approach was, to some extent, a factor in each of their assessment processes. The first utilized *only* the problem solving approach, having considered the examination complete once a problem list was identified; there was no regard for contributing factors, nor any appreciation for the patient as a whole person. The second clinician moved beyond a simple problem solving approach, showing evidence of prospective reasoning; they were able to recognize a clinical pattern which identified a segmental dysfunction as the primary source of the patient's symptoms. However, this clinician did not take note of other factors which would have affected their overall ability to successfully *manage* this patient. The third clinician, working from a sound clinical reasoning perspective, identified all the factors and issues at work in this patient's presentation and came to the most reasoned decision regarding management.

Prospective clinical reasoning involves a sophisticated analytical process utilized by clinicians in the formation of an accurate diagnosis and prognosis and in the development of a sound management plan. The overall goal of the prospective clinical reasoning model is to obtain as clear an understanding as possible of the patient's fundamental neuromusculoskeletal dysfunction, as well as any other factors which might affect the clinical management of the patient.

By itself, the problem solving model attempts only to identify the various problems encountered by the patient. Furthermore, implicit in the problem solving approach is the idea that the clinician becomes responsible for solving the patient's problems. A patient may present with neuromusculoskeletal pathology which is not amenable to physiotherapeutic management, or they may have other issues which make it unlikely that physiotherapeutic intervention will be successful. In the situation where the patient's primary dysfunction is not amenable to either conservative or surgical intervention, it may be appropriate to manage the patient from a problem solving perspective in an effort to improve their quality of life. Well developed clinical reasoning abilities allow the clinician to determine which component of the patient's presentation is amenable to physiotherapeutic management and to develop the most appropriate management plan.

Summary

The segmental dysfunction model, with its foundations in prospective clinical reasoning and an evidence-based proposal of the pathomechanics of lumbar spine pathology, provides several opportunities for the clinician to objectively assess and monitor the patient who presents with symptoms secondary to lumbar dysfunction. As will be seen, it is possible to develop a clinical appreciation for segmental and regional stiffness and the performance of the active subsystem. This permits the clinician to develop a great deal more confidence in their initial diagnosis and prognosis, as well as in their ongoing assessment of the patient's response to treatment. Furthermore, this improved ability to appreciate the extent of the segmental dysfunction associated with given patient's presentation allows for the provision of a more effective and predictable model of clinical management.

assessment of lumbar segmental dysfunction

This chapter details the structure of, and underlying rationale for, a comprehensive neuromusculo-skeletal examination of the patient who presents with suspected lumbar dysfunction. While some clinicians will be familiar with much of the material, it is anticipated that even these readers will find something new here; either a technical point, an interpretive concept or a philosophical perspective. Other readers, for example students or clinicians without a significant background in either orthopaedics or manual therapy, will find this material novel almost in its entirety.

The Subjective Examination

CLINICAL REASONING BEGINS when the clinician first observes the new patient as they enter the assessment room and continues throughout the subjective and objective examination. During the subjective examination the clinician should attempt to answer the following questions:

Is the patient's dysfunction most likely to be of visceral, peripheral neuromusculoskeletal, spinal neuromusculoskeletal or psychosocial origin?

- is there a peripheral or spinal mechanism which may be perpetuating their primary dysfunction?
- is there an affective (psychological) component to the patient's symptom presentation?
- is there an absence of evidence suggestive of neuromusculoskeletal dysfunction and/or evidence of a visceral origin for the patient's complaint?

As the patient is directed through the subjective examination, the clinician actively attempts to determine whether the patient's symptoms arise from some peripheral structure, a spinal structure, or whether they involve the central sensitization of a pain state. In some cases, patients will present with a combination of all of the above. In others, the history will lack any evidence of neuromusculo-

74

skeletal dysfunction and may instead offer evidence suggestive of systemic or visceral pathology. Answering these questions is an essential first step in focusing the clinician on the next phase of the reasoning process.

Is there any need for special tests or any reason to suspect ominous systemic pathology?

The patient may describe symptoms which prompt the clinician to perform additional safety tests. This additional testing may include, for example, a complete neurological examination, cranial nerve screening, or upper motor neuron lesion testing. It is likely that at least once in the clinician's career, a patient will report a set of symptoms which prompt the clinician to deliver the patient *via* ambulance to the local emergency department.

Is the patient describing a mechanical or an inflammatory cause for their symptoms?

The clinician should determine if the patient's symptoms are the result of an inflammatory process, some form of mechanical dysfunction, or both. This is helpful in deciding whether anti-inflammatory modalities will be truly therapeutic for the patient's symptoms. If the patient's symptoms are primarily mechanical, modalities will be of little benefit. There are a number of clues which will help the clinician in this regard.

- have anti-inflammatory medications been helpful?
- if the patient reports increased symptoms with static postures, does any change in position significantly reduce their symptoms? (this suggests a mechanical cause for their symptoms)
- is there a prolonged period of stiffness? (this suggests an inflammatory component to the patient's symptoms)

The clinician must weigh the evidence in the subjective examination which would confirm or

negate their mechanical/inflammatory pain hypothesis. In almost every case there is some amount of conflicting evidence to consider.

What is the irritability of the patient's condition? Does this indicate caution in terms of the tests selected for the physical examination?

Irritability refers to the degree of load or tissue stress required to generate symptoms relative to the length of time the symptoms subsequently persist. If minimal insult is required to increase the patient's symptoms for an extended period, their condition is said to be highly irritable. If prolonged and strenuous activity increases a patient's symptoms for only a brief period, their condition is said to be only mildly irritable. The patient with a highly irritable condition should be assessed with caution in terms of the objective tests selected. Tests which place only a low load on spinal tissues should be used on initial assessment. The patient with a mildly irritable condition can reasonably be expected to tolerate more stressful testing without significant aggravation.

What tests should be performed to confirm or negate the clinician's suspicions as to the spinal segment(s) responsible for the patient's symptoms?

As the clinician is developing their differential diagnosis, they should also be selecting the tests to be used to confirm their suspected diagnosis. The clinician should test for those segments which might be directly associated with the patient's symptoms, as well as those which might be expected to maintain or perpetuate the patient's dysfunction. Determining the answers to these questions tremendously improves the clinician's ability to form a valid diagnosis, establish an accurate prognosis and develop an effective management plan for their patient. The precise methods by which the clinician arrives at answers for these questions varies from patient to patient and will likely vary between clinicians as well.

As treatment is initiated, the clinician should monitor or re-assess the patient's response to treatment. The diagnosis is substantiated only when the patient responds as predicted to the treatment plan. If the patient does not respond as predicted, the clinician must re-assess the patient to determine the reason for this deviation from the predicted course of recovery.

It is important to note that in certain instances the subjective examination will not yield any form of clinical pattern typical for neuromusculoskeletal dysfunction. In such situations, there may or may not be evidence of systemic pathology or marked psychosocial dysfunction. In the case where no recognizable neuromusculoskeletal pattern is noted yet there is also a lack of evidence for other mechanisms, the clinician is required to perform a retrospective examination; that is, ask all questions, perform all known tests then review the data and attempt to identify any clinical pattern which may or may not be present.

History of the Present Problem

THE FINDINGS FROM the subjective examination must provide the clinician with a detailed understanding of the patient's symptoms, sufficient to form a differential diagnosis. An accurate understanding of the patient's condition is rarely developed based on their answers to one or two questions. Instead, it is the clinician's ability to identify relationships between a number of factors, both subjective and objective, that leads to a reasonable diagnosis and prognosis. Key issues to explore include:

- causation
- duration
- progression over time
- aggravating and easing factors
- irritability
- time of day influences
- location
- pain quality
- past medical and injury history

- effects of common medications
- the patient's perception of their dysfunction and expectations of treatment

Causation

The clinician must determine if the patient's symptoms are of traumatic, sudden or insidious onset. If sudden, was there a traumatic event and if so, how significant were the forces involved? It is reasonable to presume that a more or less direct relationship exists between the magnitude of the forces involved in a traumatic injury and the degree of sustained tissue damage (McGill, 2002c). Recall that not all sudden onset symptoms are related to trauma. While there is generally a relationship between the severity of trauma and the extent of the resulting pathology, some problems of 'non-traumatic' origin can be quite impressive in terms of their severity. The patient who experiences sudden, excruciating back and leg pain as they get out of bed in the morning has not experienced *trauma* in the conventional sense. Nonetheless, this historical information combined with findings from the objective physical exam, may indicate a patient who has sustained significant disruption of a variety of osseoligamentous structures at a lumbar motion segment.

Patients who present with gradual onset or sudden yet non-traumatic histories are increasingly common in the authors' clinical practices. It is essential that clinicians appreciate that such presentations may arise *via* a wide variety of mechanisms. Biomechanical motion faults, inflammatory systemic conditions, infection and neoplasm should each be considered as possible diagnoses in patients lacking an obvious mechanism of injury. The clinician must consider the relationships between a variety of subjective and objective factors in order to distinguish those patients whose symptoms are secondary to some form of neuromusculoskeletal dysfunction from those who must be referred to their family physician.

Duration and Progression

The clinician must determine how long the patient's current symptoms have been present and whether there is a trend toward improvement, whether the symptoms are worsening or whether they have become static. This provides some insight into the nature of the problem, and more information regarding the prognosis. Generally, problems with a recent onset which are showing a trend toward improvement will have a better prognosis. Symptoms which are worsening over time may indicate a more severe condition and/or a patient whose neuromuscular system is no longer able to compensate for their dysfunction. Either way, such presentations typically have a poorer prognosis. Symptoms which remain fairly static over time may indicate a problem perpetuated by some combination of habitual activity and biomechanical dysfunction adjacent to the primary lesion.

Patients with long standing conditions should be more accurately identified as having either chronic or episodic histories. The patient who has chronic low back pain (i.e., they have had symptoms most days of the week, every week for at least six months) is typically more challenging to treat. However, their prognosis should not necessarily be expected to be poor. Outcomes studies of interventions which include therapeutic segmental stabilization exercises emphasizing motor re-education of muscles such as transversus abdominis and multifidus have been shown to be effective in recurrent and/or chronic low back pain populations (O'Sullivan et al., 1997; Brox et al., 2003; Niemisto et al., 2003; Shaughnessy & Caulfield, 2004).

Occasionally, the patient with a long history begins to describe in detail several decades of back pain experience; the clinician must focus such patients upon the current episode. While knowledge of the patient's previous history in general is necessary from a prognostic perspective, it is far more important from a diagnostic and management perspective to determine the salient features of the current episode. The current episode may or may not be directly related to the patient's previous history. The clinician, through careful questioning, must make this determination.

Symptom Aggravating and Easing Factors

The clinician should ask the open ended question, "What have you noticed that makes your typical pain either worse or better?" From there, the clinician should look for specific relationships between increases and decreases in the patient's symptoms and clinically relevant factors such as rest versus activity, weightbearing versus non-weightbearing, flexion versus extension and time-of-day influences. Back pain which is due to segmental instability is often alleviated by frequent changes in static posture or gentle physical activity such as walking. More significant instabilities are often quite unpredictable in terms of the activities which elicit symptoms. Conditions which are primarily inflammatory in origin (chemically mediated) may remain just as symptomatic at rest as they are with activity. However, even the patient with chemically mediated symptoms will typically describe some degree of symptom modification of a mechanical nature.

Pain which is worsened by prolonged static postures may be due to the mechanical deformation of connective tissues which develops secondary to creep. It is thought that when a patient's symptoms are attributable to creep, their symptoms will likely be longer lasting and may not be quickly alleviated with changes in position. Furthermore, the patient will often report a prolonged period of stiffness following a period of static positioning if their symptoms are related to the effects of creep.

When considering aggravating and easing factors, the clinician must be cautious in ensuring that they have an accurate understanding of the mechanics involved. While sitting is typically considered to be a flexion dominant, weight-bearing posture, some patients learn to sit with their lumbar spine in extension. Some learn to subtly shift their weight when sitting in order to unload the symptomatic segment. Such patients may state that they have no pain while sitting since they do not recognize or recall that they have adopted these accommodative practices.

Many clinicians have been taught to look for associations between flexion or extension postures and the patient's symptoms in order to identify either disc or zygapophysial pathology. In reality, determining the direction of movement that tends to aggravate the patient's typical pain has little capacity to accurately identify the involved structure (MacNab, 1971). Rather, it identifies the direction of segmental motion which exacerbates the patient's symptoms (O'Sullivan, 2000). For example, the patient whose symptoms are consistently aggravated by lumbar extension has a form of segmental dysfunction which is either aggravated by extension of the involved segment or by the extension of an adjacent segment.

Irritability

Determining the irritability of the patient's dysfunction aids in the development of both the objective examination as well as the initial treatment plan. A patient's condition is deemed highly irritable if a relatively minor load, applied across the dysfunctional segment, results in a prolonged exacerbation of their symptoms. Alternatively, a patient's condition is considered to be of minimal irritability if a relatively brief exacerbation is elicited with significant loading of the dysfunctional segment. During the subjective examination, the identification of a highly irritable condition should preclude the use of more aggressive mechanical testing as this would significantly and unnecessarily aggravate the patient's symptoms. Assessment of the patient with an irritable lesion should involve only low load tests of limited duration. Conversely, if the patient's condition is deemed to be of low irritability, testing may be more aggressive and may be repeated as needed in order to obtain a clear understanding of the patient's dysfunction.

The clinician should recall that irritability is not strongly related to severity. A condition can result in severe pain and be of minimal or low irritability. Consider the patient who experiences sharp and severe low back pain with trunk flexion but is symptom free once they have returned to upright standing. This presentation would suggest a high severity of symptoms albeit with very low irritability; their symptoms were severe but not long lasting.

Time of Day Influences

The patient's typical pattern of symptom behaviour across the day should also be established. Are the patient's symptoms worse in the morning (suggestive of an inflammatory mechanism) or at the end of the day (suggestive of a mechanical mechanism)? An understanding of this will assist the clinician in terms of both diagnosis and management. Do they tend to have more pain late at night or do they have pain which wakes them from sleep? Is there no such pattern? The situation where a patient's symptoms are increased at the end of their relatively sedentary work day yet they report less severe symptoms throughout their active weekend is interesting. Is there something physical (static positioning) or non-physical (stress) about their work which is affecting their condition? Time-of-day changes are of particular interest to a clinician attempting to assess a patient in the morning when their symptoms typically manifest only at the end of a day's work.

Location

Whenever possible, the clinician must identify the exact location of the patient's symptoms. Specific questioning is used to determine if the patient's symptoms are dermatomal, radicular (suggestive of specific nerve root irritation) or radiating (secondary to peripheral nerve irritation). Clinically, diffuse symptoms, for example along the anterior thigh, are considered to be dermatomal in origin. Radicular and radiating pain are suggestive of either chemical or mechanical compromise of the conductive elements of the nervous tissues, a spinal nerve root in the case of radicular pain, or a peripheral nerve in the case of radiating pain. Both radicular and radiating symptoms may serve as clinical indicators of more severe pathology. The specific pattern of the patient's symptoms is useful for the clinician as the location and path of a referred or radiating symptom may suggest a dysfunctional segment in the lumbar spine.

Those patients who present with symptoms restricted to the lower extremity are of particular interest to the authors. In our opinion, while peripheral symptoms secondary to a recent traumatic event are almost always indicative of peripheral pathology, peripheral symptoms which develop without a history of trauma and in an otherwise healthy individual are often representative of lumbar segmental dysfunction with referral to the lower extremity (see case study 2, page 143). In some cases, true peripheral pathology may develop as a result of the neuromuscular dysfunction which develops in the presence of a segmental dysfunction in the lumbar spine (see case study 1, page 141). Finally, peripheral symptoms which persist or re-appear long after a traumatic peripheral injury may indicate a local injury to the peripheral nervous system. Trauma in the periphery may result in impaired neurodynamics at the initial injury site. Complex clinical presentations, featuring a variety of lower extremity symptoms, can arise when combined lumbar and peripheral lesions lead to a 'double-crush' syndrome. In such cases it may be argued that the nervous system itself becomes pathological and is the generator of the patient's pain and swelling (Daemen et al., 1998).

Clinically, there is often little correlation between the severity of the patient's dysfunction and the extent to which their symptoms remain localized to the lumbar spine. This may be due, at least in part, to the multi-dimensional nature of the pain experience. Although symptoms which are restricted to the lumbar spine are often considered suggestive of less severe neuro-musculoskeletal dysfunction, symptoms which extend into the lower extremity may or may not indicate more extensive segmental pathology. A variety of pain features including intensity, quality and distribution may vary without any change in the severity of the patient's primary neuromusculoskeletal dysfunction.

Pain Quality

Clinically, there appears to be some correlation between certain pain descriptors and the nature of the patient's dysfunction. However, clinicians should bear in mind that people vary in terms of their subjective interpretation of their own symptoms as well as in their ability to adequately verbalize these sensations. The patient's report of symptoms can be influenced by factors which may not be related to the extent of their injury and include such things as beliefs about pain, cultural influences, fear, stress, and their immune system status (Butler & Moseley, 2003). The clinician should appreciate that while such descriptors may occasionally provide information regarding the likely region of dysfunction, they are generally of little value in determining the specific structure at fault.

Two descriptors which do seem to correlate well with the nature of the patient's dysfunction are 'burning pain' and 'intense, flash-like' or 'sharp pain'. 'Burning' pain is very often indicative of neurogenic involvement, whereas low back pain described as sharp, intense and transient is typical of significant mechanical dysfunction. 'Dull', 'aching', or 'diffuse' are terms frequently associated with a variety of problems, and therefore these descriptions tend to be less powerful diag-nostically. Similarly, the patient's description of their pain intensity is often poorly indicative of the severity of their pathology. This feature of the pain experience seems especially related to affective function (and thus dysfunction) and is best used as an indicator of the extent to which a patient perceives their condition to be changing during treatment.

Past Medical and Injury History

Enquiring as to the patient's medical and injury history provides prognostic information as well as information which may be used to guide management. As part of the initial subjective examination, the clinician should determine:

- if the patient's overall health may be expected to limit their rate or potential for recovery
- if the patient's history includes any systemic disease states which demand that certain interventions be applied with caution or others to be considered as contraindicated
- if the patient has sustained any previous injury which might be related to their current presentation

For example, diabetes mellitus has been shown to significantly reduce the potential for healing in patients with any form of injury. Similarly, a patient's prognosis should be modified if it were found that they had experienced a ten year history of lower quadrant symptoms secondary to a severe trauma. A medical history which includes osteoporosis would prompt the clinician to consider certain mobilization and/or manipulative techniques to be contraindicated.

Effects of Common Medications

There are many types of medication which are typically prescribed for the patient with low back pain. These include muscle relaxants, non-steroidal anti-inflammatory's (NSAIDs) and analgesics. The patient's response to some of these medications may assist the clinician in determining the type of pain with which the patient presents. For example, if the patient responds well to NSAIDs, the clinician can rationally expect that the patient's symptoms are related to an inflammatory process. If NSAID's are ineffective, the patient's symptoms are more likely mechanical in origin rather than chemical or inflammatory.

The Patient's Perception of their Dysfunction and Expectations of Treatment

This information is extremely useful to the clinician, yet in our experience as educators, few clinicians seek to understand this feature of their patient's presentation. In the presence of mild to moderate neuromusculoskeletal pathology, if the patient's perception of the severity of their dysfunction is one of severe and permanent dysfunction, the likelihood of achieving any sort of meaningful treatment outcome is limited. In such situations, the patient's perception can limit their compliance with any treatment approach due to fear of exacerbation of symptoms and further regression of their underlying condition. An alternate scenario involves the patient who believes that they must endure a significant amount of pain in order to recover. In both cases the prognosis is seriously compromised.

A patient's perceptions, both adaptive and maladaptive, are influenced by a number of factors. The patient's prior history of injury, the results of various diagnostic tests, even their interactions with family, friends, health professionals, lawyers and insurance company representatives, can influence their perception of the current condition. While neuromusculoskeletal clinicians are certainly not trained to manage such issues, they must be aware of the potential for such psychosocial factors to affect the patient's perception of their condition. As described in chapter four, the Roland-Morris Disability Questionnaire and the Oswestry Disability Questionnaire have been reported as being valid, reliable and efficient tools for assessing a patient's self-perceived level of disability (Roland & Fairbank, 2000).

The goals of the patient's management approach must be established during the initial examination. This is important from the clinician's perspective as the patient may have unrealistic expectations of treatment in terms of timeframe and/or final outcome. Identifying such issues early rather than later avoids the unfortunate situation where a patient expects to be symptom free following two treatment sessions, while the clinician does not expect to see any significant changes in symptoms for six to eight visits. If such unrealistic expectations are identified early, the clinician can hopefully help the patient establish more realistic expectations. If this cannot be achieved, appropriate management may involve referral of the patient for a second opinion.

The Objective Examination

Active Range of Motion Tests

This should be conducted with the patient in the position which most easily exacerbates their symptoms, whether this occurs in sitting or standing, or during a particular phase of the gait cycle. The clinician must keep in mind that they are searching for movement asymmetries in the lumbar spine - regions or segments that appear to move too little or too much. The assessment of the lumbar spine should not be an exercise in simple symptom provocation.

Standing AROM

The patient is standing with equal weight on each foot and both knees extended (a standardized start position). Movements from this standing start position should be performed in order from least to most provocative. Flexion and extension are best observed from an oblique angle, with the clinician slightly behind and to the side of the patient (figure 5.1). Sidebending is best observed from directly behind the patient (figure 5.2).

Occasionally these movements should be tested with the patient initiating the movement from the pelvis rather than the trunk. Flexion and extension may be initiated 'from below' by asking the patient to perform a pelvic tilt, either posteriorly or anteriorly (figure 5.3). Sidebending can be initiated 'from below' by flexing one knee. For example, right sidebending 'from below' is tested by having the patient flex their left knee, resulting in a relative right sidebend through the lumbar spine (figure 5.4). Movements tested 'from below' are especially useful when testing the L5-S1 motion segment. It is believed that movements from below require the patient to move through the lumbosacral junction and subsequently load any dysfunctional structures around this segment. When movements of the trunk are initiated from above it is thought that the patient may modify their movements to minimize the load at the dysfunctional lumbosacral junction. These compensations may go unnoticed by the clinician resulting in false negatives on AROM testing.

The clinician should observe not only the quantity of movement but more importantly the quality of the movement. Is there a 'stutter' noted through the lumbar spine with the movement? Is there a lateral shift or translation evident through sidebending? How does the patient arrive at their

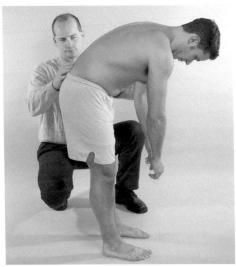
Figure 5.1 Observation of active lumbar flexion.

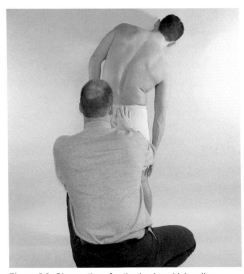
Figure 5.2 Observation of active lumbar sidebending.

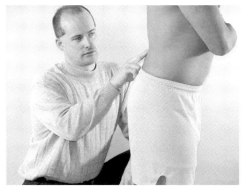

Figure 5.3 Lumbar extension tested 'from below' as the patient actively rotates their pelvis anteriorly.

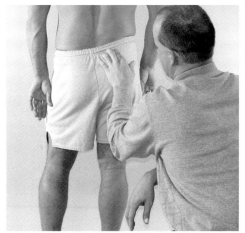

Figure 5.4 Relative right side flexion of the lumbar spine tested 'from below' *via* active left knee flexion.

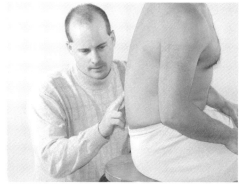

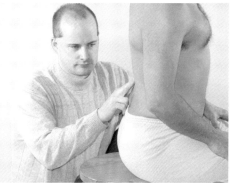

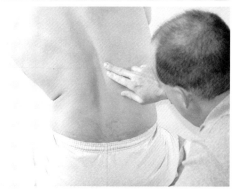

Figure 5.5a,b,c. Seated AROM testing: flexion (posterior pelvic tilting); extension (anterior pelvic tilting); and side flexion.

end position? The clinician should note how the movement affects the patient's symptoms throughout range. Useful questions to ask are "what stopped you from moving further?" and "how does this movement change your symptoms?" Active movements may be overpressured if minimal symptoms are present.

Seated AROM

The patient who notes that their symptoms are exacerbated in sitting should be assessed in sitting. With the patient in a seated position, flexion in the lumbar region is checked by asking the patient to sit back on their sacrum or roll their pelvis backwards (figure 5.5a). Extension is attained by asking the patient to then roll forward on their 'sitting' bones or stick their backside out (figure 5.5b). Sidebending is achieved by having the patient maintain an equal amount of weight through both ischial tuberosities as they bring their shoulder 'through the trunk' towards the opposite hip (figure 5.5c). This can be further facilitated by placing a rolled towel under the buttock ipsilateral to the direction of sidebending being tested. Again, these may be overpressured if minimal symptoms are noted.

Gait-biased AROM

Patients who have more symptoms during gait should be assessed while in a walking stance (figure 5.6). The patient is asked to stand as if in mid-stance, first with the left and then the right as the forward limb. In each posture they should rock back and forth while the clinician notes quantity, quality and symmetry of spinal AROM.

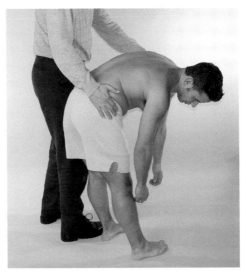

Figure 5.7 The patient is guided through a combination of flexion and right side bending.

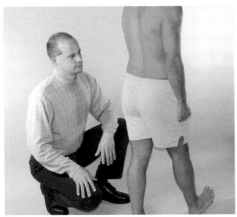

Figure 5.6 Start position for observation of gait-biased AROM assessment with a patient who reports symptoms at the moment of right initial contact. From this posture, the patient moves through the cardinal planes of lumbar movement.

Combined Movement Tests

COMBINED MOVEMENT TESTS are performed when the cardinal plane AROM tests are relatively unremarkable and generate only minimal symptoms. By performing active movements in this manner, greater compressive and tensile forces are applied to the lumbar spine. Combined movement testing allows the clinician to determine whether a patient with relatively normal cardinal plane AROM is limited into one of the primary 'quadrants' of the lumbar spine.

The four combined movement positions tested are flexion plus left sidebending, flexion plus right sidebending, extension plus left sidebending, and extension plus right sidebending (figures 5.7 and 5.8). As with AROM tests, the quality of movement is as important as the quantity of movement.

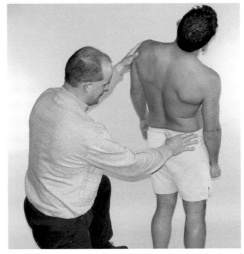

Figure 5.8 The patient is guided through a combination of extension and right side bending.

These movements may be over pressured if minimal symptoms are noted. Often a difference in end-feel is noted by the clinician before the patient reports a change in their symptoms.

The 'H & I' Test

THE 'H&I' TEST IS USED to elicit further information regarding the biomechanical nature of a patient's limitation into one of the four quadrants or combined movements as described in the previous section. Clinically it has been observed that the sequencing of the components of the combined movements can affect the patient's available range of motion into a quadrant in addition to the symptoms noted by the patient at the end of their available range. For example, on combined movement testing a patient with lumbar dysfunction is noted to be limited and mildly symptomatic into the right extension quadrant if they extend first and then add right sidebending. However, it is noted that if the patient performs right sidebending before extending, they are no longer limited in range and their symptoms are minimal.

This clinical observation may be accounted for by one or both (or neither) of two hypotheses. The first is based on Fryette's 3rd law of spinal motion and is in keeping with the tri-planar model of lumbar segmental motion. In the above example, the tri-planar model would suggest that the dysfunctional segment experiences an excess amount of connective tissue compliance or 'give' along a translation in the sagittal plane as the patient extends their lumbar spine. If the patient extends first, they move into the direction of their clinical instability and reproduce their symptoms. From this position of dysfunctional extension, the segment is unable to move fully into sidebending. However, if the patient initiates the combined movement with sidebending (a movement in the coronal plane which, theoretically, should not be influenced by clinical instability in the sagittal plane) the segment is effectively stabilized through a 'pre-tensioning' of the passive elements of the motion segment. This pre-tensioning is thought to limit the amount of sagittal plane translation available at the segment and as a result the patient is able to complete the quadrant more fully.

A competing and more current hypothesis states that in moving into the dysfunctional position, an excessive amount of compensatory multi-segmental muscle contraction is developed which alters the dysfunctional segment's axis of rotation. This protective but excessive contraction limits the dysfunctional segment from moving fully into the sidebending position. If the patient moves first into sidebending, they in effect avoid their dysfunctional position (in this case, pure extension)

and avoid triggering the compensatory, protective muscle contraction. As such, they move more fully into the extension quadrant.

The H & I test is performed with the patient standing with equal weight on each foot and their knees extended. This will effectively localize the motion to the spine rather than, *via* compensation, through the lower limbs. The 'H' component is performed by having the patient sidebend as fully as possible, followed by either flexion or extension. The 'I' component of the test begins with either flexion or extension to the patient's available limit, followed by the sidebending movements. Practically, each quadrant should be tested, and each pathway within each quadrant examined and compared. Figure 5.9 describes the H & I test graphically.

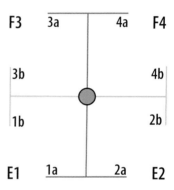

Figure 5.9 The H & I test described schematically. The 'H' pathway is shown in light gray; its pathways are identified as 1b, 2b, 3b and 4b. The 'I' pathway is shown in dark gray; its pathways are identified as 1a, 2a, 3a and 4a. Whereas the standard combined movement test compares movement into the two extension quadrants (E1 and E2) and into the two flexion quadrants (F3 and F4) the H & I test considers the symmetry of motion into each quadrant via two different pathways; thus, we are testing for the symmetry of E1a vs E1b, E2a vs E2b, F3a vs F3b and F4a vs F4b. For example, the final position of E1 is attained via pathways 1b and 1a. Ideally, pathways 1a and 1b attain the same E1 and thus E1a = E1b. If E1a is notably different from E1b, an asymmetrical limitation of motion into the quadrant is noted and is considered suggestive of clinical instability or segmental dysfunction.

Typically, patients with lumbar dysfunction exhibit either a symmetrical or asymmetrical pattern of restriction on H & I testing. A symmetrical limitation into any one quadrant will thus be identical to the findings on combined movement testing. An asymmetrical limitation into any single quadrant occurs when the patient's final position into the quadrant varies depending on which movement is performed first. Clinically, this asymmetry is interpreted as being strongly suggestive of at least a moderate degree of clinical instability or segmental dysfunction.

Passive Segmental Tests

PASSIVE SEGMENTAL TESTS are used to evaluate the quality and quantity of movement in the lumbar spine at a segmental level. The clinician should pay close attention to the amount of connective tissue tension that may be applied across the segment prior to the onset of symptoms; this data is invaluable in determining the irritability of the patient's condition.

Passive Intervertebral Movement Testing

Passive intervertebral movement (PIVM) testing is used to determine the quantity and quality of passive physiological movement available at a motion segment. Such tests of intervertebral range of motion are analogous to passive range of motion testing at peripheral joints. It is important for the clinician to note the onset of tension or stiffness relative to the overall segmental range as well as where in the range any symptoms are reproduced.

Interestingly, Maitland's concept of the movement diagram demonstrates that manual therapists have been monitoring neutral zone:elastic zone relationships for decades. Maitland used the movement diagram to chart the mechanical behaviour of joints on assessment and during treatment (figure 5.10). Maitland's R1 is synonymous with the boundary between the NZ and EZ while R2 represents the anatomical limit of motion at the joint, or the outer limit of the EZ.

Segmental Compliance Testing

At the end of the segment's range (R2), the clini-

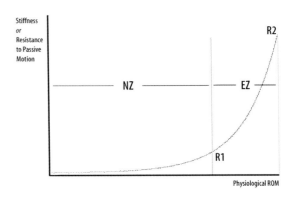

Figure 5.10 Maitland's movement diagram superimposed with Panjabi's NZ:EZ model of stiffness behaviour across the physiological range of motion. It is proposed that the boundary between the NZ and the EZ corresponds with the point where a sharp increase in resistance to passive motion is first appreciated *via* a manual therapy examination.

cian determines the 'end feel' for that movement. The term 'end feel' refers to the degree of segmental stiffness or connective tissue compliance at the position of R2. Since the joint is assessed for 'end feel' at the end of its physiological ROM, 'end feel' should not be construed as involving any amount of movement of the motion segment. The joint is already at its R2, there is no further movement possible. Rather, 'end feel' refers to the quantity and quality of connective tissue compliance at R2.

Traditionally, the term Passive Accessory Intervertebral Movement (PAIVM) has been applied to this component of the segmental biomechanical examination. However, in the authors' opinion, PAIVM is an unfortunate term, as it implies that the clinician is attempting to appreciate some amount of motion. Indeed, many students find these tests confusing from a conceptual and thus an interpretive perspective, as they assume from the test's name that they are looking for movement of some form. Rather than assessing for movement, PAIVM tests are intended to assess the segmental stiffness or connective tissue compliance of the arthrokinematic motions associated with the various physiological movements of the segment. The clinician is attempting to appreciate the degree of compliance or 'give' present in the connective tissues when the segment is at its R2. The traditional terms used to describe 'end feel' reflect the subjective nature of the test; end feels have been described as *bone-to-bone, spasm, capsular, springy block, tissue approximation, and empty* (Cyriax, 1982).

Since the term PAIVM is inherently problematic, we have developed the term *Segmental Compliance Test* (SCT) and have used this terminology throughout this text. Practically, both PIVMs and SCTs are selected based on the results of the patient's AROM examination. The clinician would typically assess the PIVM associated with whichever active movement was most limited and the SCT associated with the PIVM which was most dysfunctional. For example, if flexion was most limited on active movement testing, the flexion PIVM would be tested first, followed by the appropriate SCT for that PIVM.

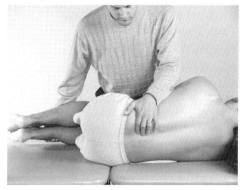

Figure 5.11 Flexion PIVM - clinician and patient positioning. Note the towel placed under the patient to reduce the degree of lumbar sidebending; this is most necessary with patients who have broad shoulders or broad pelvises.

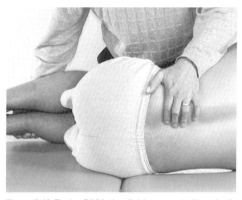

Figure 5.12 Flexion PIVM - the clinician supports the patient's lower limbs via their anterior hip and caudal hand. The amount and quality of passive flexion is appreciated by palpation of the interspinous interval.

Flexion Tests

Flexion PIVM
The patient is side-lying in the center of the plinth with their hips and knees flexed. The clinician's caudal arm and hand supports the patient's lower extremities against the clinicians hip so that the clinician can maneuver the patient's lower extremities. The clinician then guides the patient's lower extremities anteriorly along the plinth creating a progressive lumbar flexion (figure 5.11). The clinician palpates the interspinous space of the segment being evaluated with the cranial hand while creating lumbar flexion through the patient's lower extremities with their caudal upper limb (figure 5.12). The clinician attempts to appreciate the relative amount of flexion at each lumbar segment.

Clinical Tip:
If the patient has difficulty relaxing during passive segmental testing the clinician may use their upper body to lightly compress the patient's lower limbs against the plinth. This will often enable the patient to relax, allowing passive testing to proceed more effectively.

Flexion SCT
The clinician brings the segment to the end of its available flexion range using a typical PIVM. To assess the segmental compliance associated with the arthrokinematics of flexion, the clinician, using their caudal hand, performs a P-A pressure directed cranially on the inferior aspect of the spinous process of the superior vertebrae of the motion segment (figure 5.13). This SCT simultaneously assesses the connective tissue compliance or 'give' associated with the posterior to anterior rock at the interbody joint and the bilateral superior and anterior slide at the z-joints.

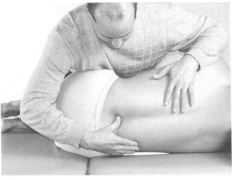

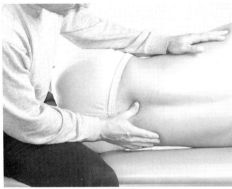

Figure 5.13 Flexion SCT - the clinician applies a cranially directed posterior-anterior force at the inferior aspect of the **superior** vertebrae of the motion segment with the segment positioned at the end of its available flexion range. In the bottom photo, the clinician is seated behind the patient - some clinicians may find this a more efficient position from which to apply this technique.

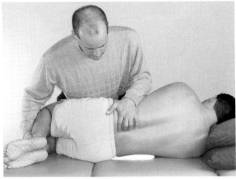

Figure 5.14 Extension PIVM - clinician and patient positioning. The patient is positioned towards the near edge of the plinth; their knees are flexed to facilitate lumbar extension by tensioning the rectus femoris and thus anteriorly rotating the pelvis.

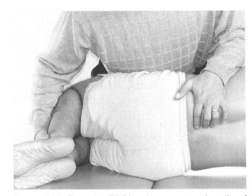

Figure 5.15 Extension PIVM - the amount and quality of passive extension generated *via* the clinician's caudal hand is appreciated by palpation of the interspinous interval at each lumbar motion segment using the clinician's cranial hand.

Extension Tests

Extension PIVM

The patient assumes a side-lying posture towards the near edge of the plinth. The patient's knees are then fully flexed by the clinician's caudal arm and hand with the clinician's cranial hand palpating the interspinous space of the segment being evaluated. The flexion of the patient's knees is thought to increase tension in the rectus femoris, thereby facilitating extension of the lumbar spine, as the pelvis is drawn into a more anteriorly rotated position. The clinician then guides the patient's lower extremities posteriorly along the plinth creating a progressive lumbar extension (figure 5.14). The amount of this passive extension is palpated using the cranial hand at each lumbar motion segment (figure 5.15).

Extension SCT

The clinician performs a PIVM and brings the segment to the end of available extension. One might assume that to assess the segmental compliance associated with the arthrokinematics of *extension* at both the interbody and the z-joints, the clinician could simply use a P-A pressure directed caudally on the spinous process of the superior vertebrae of the motion segment, the opposite of what one does to simulate the arthrokinematics of flexion. However, this is often difficult to do. The more feasible solution is to apply a P-A pressure directed *cranially* on the inferior aspect of the spinous process of the inferior vertebrae of the motion segment (figure 5.16).

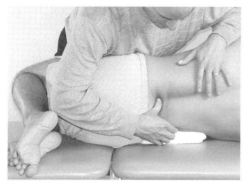

Figure 5.16 Extension SCT - the clinician applies a cranially directed posterior-anterior force at the inferior aspect of the **inferior** vertebrae of the motion segment with the segment positioned at the end of its available extension range. This is thought to create a relative extension at the target segment.

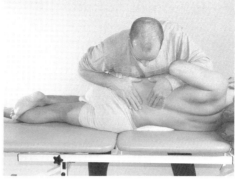

Figure 5.17 Sidebending/Rotation PIVM - the patient is positioned near the mid-portion of the plinth with their legs offset to encourage rotation. Folded towels are utilized to facilitate sidebending. In this example, the clinician is preparing to assess right sidebending with left rotation.

Sidebending/Rotation Tests

Sidebending/Rotation PIVM

Clinically, sidebending/rotation PIVMs are performed as part of a tri-planar PIVM involving either flexion or extension. Tri-planar PIVMs are utilized when the uniplanar (flexion or extension) AROM testing is unremarkable and combined movement testing is utilized as part of the objective exam.

The patient is asked to assume a side-lying position towards the mid-portion of the plinth. The clinician positions the target segment at its end ROM of either flexion or extension. The patient's superior lower extremity is flexed while the other is in an extended position; by offsetting the knees, the lumbar spine is more easily rotated (figure 5.17). While palpating intersegmental motion *via* the spinous processes with the cranial hand, the clinician, *via* their caudal axilla and forearm, levers the pelvis and lumbar spine into sidebending and rotation (figure 5.18).

If the patient is in right side-lying, the clinician can easily simulate and evaluate right sidebending plus left rotation via a caudal and laterally applied force through the pelvis as well as left sidebending plus left rotation *via* a cranial and medially directed force through the pelvis (the rotation evaluated, as part of a combined PIVM, is always opposite

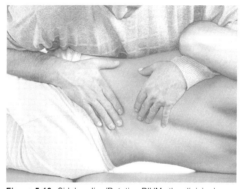

Figure 5.18 Sidebending/Rotation PIVM - the clinician's cranial hand palpates the spinous process of the segment's superior vertebra while the caudal upper extremity levers the patient's lumbar spine into right sidebending and left rotation.

to the side upon which the patient is lying).

Clinical Tip:
The position for spinal mobilization is identical to that for tri-planar PIVMs.

Sidebending/Rotation SCT
To evaluate the segmental compliance associated with the arthrokinematic motions of sidebending and rotation, the clinician positions the dysfunctional segment at the end of its available flexion or extension, side bending and rotation. The SCT is performed by applying a force through the superior spinous process of the target segment. For example, to perform the SCT for right side

bending and left rotation, the clinician positions the patient in right side lying and applies a cranial and medially directed force on the superior spinous process of the target segment (figure 5.19). For left side bending the force is directed inferiorly and medially.

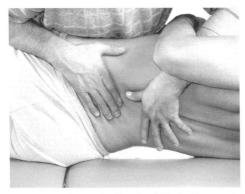

Figure 5.19 Sidebending/Rotation SCT - in this example, the clinician's left thumb applies a cranially and medially directed force from the left side of the spinous process to assess the segmental stiffness or compliance associated with right side bending and left rotation. Simultaneously, their caudal hand and forearm lever the patient's pelvis and lumbar spine into right sidebending and left rotation.

Segmental Integrity Tests (SIT)

SEGMENTAL INTEGRITY TESTS have the capacity to provide the clinician with an appreciation for the lumbar spine's stiffness or compliance characteristics, both segmentally and regionally. The extent to which a given test elicits information regarding the stiffness/compliance at a single segment likely depends upon the extent to which the load applied to the spine can be isolated to the segment of interest and thus prevented from dissipating across multiple segments. Patient positioning and the clinician's handling will therefore determine whether the test in question is more a segmental test or whether it is more of a regional test.

Tests which place greater emphasis on specific segments evaluate the ability of a motion segment's passive elements to resist uni-planar forces. They are considered to be tests of segmental stiffness or connective tissue compliance at a target motion segment in one plane of movement. As per the Panjabi model, they may also be interpreted as seg-

mental tests of the integrity of the passive subsystem, not unlike ligamentous stress testing at the knee. This type of segmental testing does not evaluate the amount of translational motion available at a motion segment. Although the amount of connective tissue 'give' or compliance at a motion segment is often confused with translational movement, it is the authors' opinion that translational segmental motion cannot be evaluated clinically, in the majority of patients. The exception would be the patient with massive disruption of the passive subsystem as seen, for example, in a grade III spondylolisthesis.

The more regional tests, those with which it is difficult to isolate our loading of the spine to a single target segment, provide the clinician with an appreciation for the stiffness/compliance characteristics of the lumbar spine when a load is applied to the spine at a certain segment and in a certain direction. Radiographic and MRI studies of the mechanical effects of tests such as the prone-lying posterior segmental integrity test (more commonly known as a posterior-anterior mobilization) confirm the absence of the traditionally anticipated anterior translation of the 'target' vertebrae as well as the regional nature of the test (Lee & Evans, 1997; Powers et al., 2003; Kulig et al., 2004; Lee et al., 2005). In the author's opinion, this important finding does not require manual therapists to abandon this nor other similar tests. However, it does necessitate major revisions regarding our interpretation of such tests in relation to the status of the lumbar spine.

Clinical Tidbit:

Both SCTs and SITs assess the compliance of the connective tissues or passive subsystem. SCTs assess the compliance of a segment's connective tissues as associated with a specific physiological movement. The SIT assesses the resulting compliance of the connective tissues when a uni-planar load is applied to the spine, either segmentally or regionally. The SITs are performed at the lumbar level identified as dysfunctional *via* the previously described PIVMs and SCTs. The relative amount of connective tissue compliance appreciated at the segment is considered to reflect the extent of any deficit of the passive elements or the passive subsystem.

Segmental Integrity vs. Stability Testing

These segmental integrity tests are historically referred to as segmental *stability* tests. At a time when the passive elements were thought to significantly control segmental motion, such terminology reflected this traditional concept of spinal function. The current evidence supports a more complex construct, with stability of the spine provided by the integrated function of the passive, active and neural control subsystems. Therefore a test of the stability of a spinal segment would need to challenge each of the three subsystems simultaneously. The segmental integrity test evaluates only the passive subsystem. While it is true that unstable segments demonstrate increased connective tissue compliance with segmental integrity testing, it is not appropriate to describe a given segment as *unstable* based solely on a test of the passive subsystem. As well as being technically incorrect, to do so will only perpetuate a state of confusion regarding current evidence-based concepts of spinal stability.

For these segmental integrity tests to be considered stability tests, the patient would need to independently activate their segmental stabilizing muscles as the clinician applied a passive uni-planar load across the segment. This form of testing could provide useful information about the neuromuscular system's potential to control uniplanar shear loads. However, from a practical perspective, such testing is difficult to utilize during the initial assessment as patients will rarely have adequate skill with such patterns of activation. Too often, on initial assessment, they will activate their multi-segmental muscles as per their typical compensatory pattern. As treatment proceeds and the patient develops greater skill with more appropriate patterns of contraction, the test may be used as a measure of the patient's progress. Assessment of the neuromuscular system is left as a separate component of the objective examination.

Panjabi hypothesized that the neural control and active subsystems could compensate for a passive subsystem deficit at an unstable lumbar motion segment (Panjabi, 1992a). This hypothesis certainly supports the use of exercise interventions as part of the management plan for patients with low back pain. Clinically, it appears that patients with low back pain of lumbar origin often present with a lumbar motion segment which has both excessive and uncontrolled motion. Therapeutic exercise programs, directed towards enhancing or restoring the function of both the active and neural control subsystems, are believed to enable the patient to achieve a measure of control over this excessive segmental motion leading to reduced pain and enhanced function. It may be necessary to consider that even in the presence of improved function of the active and neural control subsystems, both the passive subsystem deficit and the resulting excessive motion may remain despite the resolution of symptoms. The proposed improvement in the control of spinal motion is the primary goal of the exercise interventions used in this patient group.

There are five commonly utilized segmental integrity tests for the lumbar spine. These tests vary in their specificity with some being more segmental (tests 1 and 2) and others being more regional (tests 4 and 5).

1. Sidelying Anterior-Posterior Segmental Integrity Test*

The patient is positioned in side-lying with the hips flexed and the lumbar spine in neutral, close to the near edge of the plinth. The clinician stands facing the plinth and positions their lower abdomen or anterior hip (just inferomedial to the clinician's ASIS) against the patient's knees. The clinician's cranial hand palpates and fixes the superior vertebrae of the target motion segment while the caudal hand palpates the inferior vertebra's spinous process (figure 5.20). The clinician delivers a slow gradual posteriorly-directed force through the patient's thighs (figure 5.21). The clinician palpates the spinous processes of the segment to appreciate the associated connective tissue compliance or 'give' at the target segment.

*Segmental Integrity Tests are named for the direction of applied load as opposed to an assumed direction of segmental translation or movement.

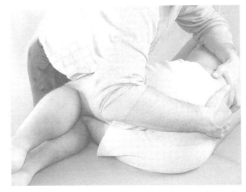

Figure 5.20 Sidelying Anterior Posterior Segmental Integrity Test - patient and clinician positioning. The clinician's lower abdomen (adjacent to the anterior superior iliac spine) supports the patient's knees. The patient is positioned towards the near edge of the plinth.

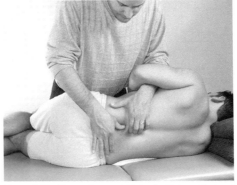

Figure 5.22 Rotary Segmental Integrity Test - patient and clinician positioning. The clinician's cranial hand fixes the superior vertebra of the target segment. A rotational force is applied to the segment's inferior vertebra through its spinous process.

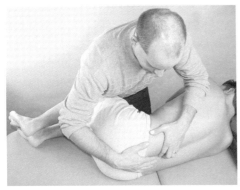

Figure 5.21 Sidelying Anterior Posterior Segmental Integrity Test. The clinician fixes the superior vertebra of the target segment with their cranial hand and applies a posteriorly directed force along the patient's thigh. The spinous process of the segment's inferior vertebra is palpated to appreciate the degree and quality of connective tissue compliance associated with the applied force.

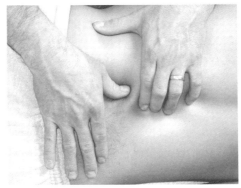

Figure 5.23 Rotary Segmental Integrity Test - clinician hand position and the direction of applied forces. The clinician's caudal hand applies a rotational force opposite to the direction of fixation applied *via* the cranial hand.

2. Rotary Segmental Integrity Test

The patient is in side-lying with the hips flexed and a neutral lumbar spine, close to the near edge of the plinth. The clinician uses their cranial hand to fix the superior vertebra of the target motion segment *via* its spinous process (figure 5.22). The clinician's caudal hand applies a rotational force to the spinous process of the inferior vertebra of the motion segment. The forces applied in the fixation of the superior vertebra and the rotation of the inferior vertebra occur in opposite directions (figure 5.23). Again, the clinician's objective is to gain an appreciation for the associated connective tissue compliance or 'give' at the target segment.

As torsional loading is controlled by the intervertebral disc, z-joints and the local musculature, it is likely that all of these structures will be dysfunctional to some degree if, in fact, excessive rotational compliance is noted at a lumbar motion segment. Therefore, if excessive connective tissue compliance is noted during a rotational segmental integrity test, it is highly likely that there is a multi-directional instability at the segment (figure 5.24). Typically, in the presence of increased compliance with a rotary SIT, one or more of the other SITs will also demonstrate increased compliance.

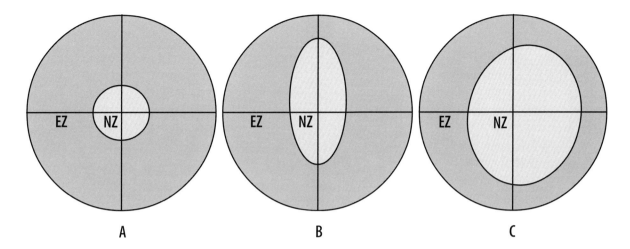

A   **B**   **C**

Figure 5.24 Hypothetical representation of the NZ:EZ:ROM relationships in normal and pathological motion segments. **A** - non-pathological motion segment. **B** - pathological segment with a markedly increased NZ, primarily through the sagittal plane. Clinically, this would be described as a uni-planar clinical instability or segmental dysfunction. **C** - pathological segment with a markedly increased NZ through more than one plane of motion. Clinically, this would be described as a multi-directional clinical instability or segmental dysfunction. A comprehensive manual therapy examination including segmental integrity testing may be capable of distinguishing between patients with uni-planar and multi-planar dysfunction. Markedly increased connective tissue compliance or 'give' with a rotary segmental integrity test is thought to be indicative of multi-planar instability.

3. Seated Anterior-Posterior Segmental Integrity Test

The patient is seated at the end of the plinth, holding a pillow against their chest with their arms folded over their anterior chest wall. The clinician stands alongside the patient, places one arm between the patient's folded arms and guides the patient into their neutral lumbar spine posture. This arm is then used to apply the posteriorly-directed force through the patient's trunk. The clinician's other hand is used to provide fixation at the motion segment to be tested (figure 5.25a). Using a modified 'pinch' grip between the thumb and D2 PIP of the free hand, the clinician fixes the inferior vertebra of the target motion segment by holding the spinous process then applies a posteriorly-directed force through the anterior trunk (figure 5.25b). *Via* this fixation hand, the clinician appreciates the associated connective tissue compliance or 'give' at the target segment.

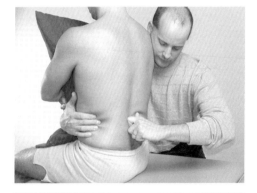

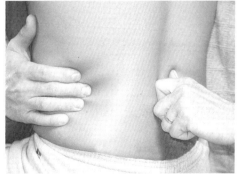

Figure 5.25 a,b   a (upper) - Seated Anterior-Posterior Segmental Integrity Test - patient and clinician positioning. **b** - clinician's hand positions; the anterior forearm applies a posteriorly-directed force while the posterior hand fixes the target segment *via* an anteriorly-directed counter force. The fixation hand monitors the segmental compliance associated with this test.

4. Prone Posterior-Anterior Segmental Integrity Test

The patient is positioned in prone lying. For comfort and to attain the patient's neutral lordosis, pillows are placed under the patient's trunk or abdomen as needed. The clinician stands directly over the target motion segment and applies an anteriorly-directed force to the inferior vertebra of the target segment (figure 5.26). Traditionally, this was believed to create a relative posterior translation at the target segment. However, as discussed previously, recent imaging studies have shown that this does not occur; instead, the spine bows into extension (Lee & Evans, 1997; Powers et al., 2003; Kulig et al., 2004; Lee et al., 2005). Thus, this more regional test provides the clinician with an appreciation for the stiffness or compliance of the lumbar region as an anteriorly-directed force is applied across different segments of the lumbar spine.

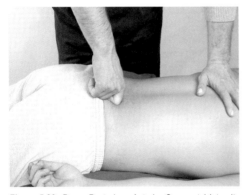

Figure 5.26 Prone Posterior - Anterior Segmental Integrity Test - patient positioning and direction of applied force. The clinician delivers an anteriorly directed force through the spinous processes of the lumbar vertebrae. A generalized increase in the lumbar lordosis occurs with this test.

5. Lateral Segmental Integrity Test

The patient is in side-lying with the hips flexed and a neutral lumbar spine, close to the near edge of the plinth. The clinician, using the ulnar border of their forearm, applies a transverse pressure to the lumbar spine (figure 5.27). With this test, the clinician is simply looking for symptom

reproduction; no degree of segmental integrity is inferred from this test. Since the test lacks specificity, it is often referred to as a stress test rather than a segmental integrity test. Relative to the sidelying anterior-posterior and rotary segmental integrity tests, this test yields only minimally useful information regarding the patient's condition.

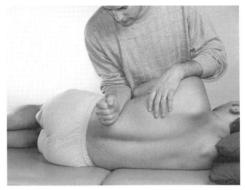

Figure 5.27 Lateral Segmental Integrity Test - patient positioning and direction of applied force. The clinician delivers a transverse force through the lateral aspect of the trunk. This is a test of symptom reproduction rather than segmental integrity and is therefore of relatively limited clinical value.

Segmental Stabilizing System Testing

IN THE THIRD CHAPTER, the lumbar active subsystem was described as consisting of the segmental stabilizing muscles (SSM) and the multi-segmental postural muscles (MPM). As reviewed previously, a range of studies have demonstrated a dysfunctional set of changes in the SSM in the presence of lumbar spine dysfunction. These changes include alterations in activation patterns of the transversus abdominis and the deep fibres of the lumbar multifidus as well as histochemical and morpohological changes in the lumbar multifidus. A segmental atrophy of the psoas muscle adjacent to an intervertebral disc herniation (Dangaria & Naesh, 1998) and ipsilateral to the symptom generating segment in patients with unilateral low back pain (Barker et al., 2004) has also been reported. Clinical tests intended to assist the clinician in appreciating certain features of this dysfunctional set have been developed.

Palpation for Segmental Lumbar Multifidus Atrophy

A SIMPLE CLINICAL TEST has been developed with which the clinician can gain an appreciation for the relative volume of the multifidus muscle. With the patient in prone lying the clinician palpates the bilateral multifidus from S1 to L2-3, comparing for symmetry of muscle volume (figure 5.28). The clinician should palpate the multifidus approximately 1.5 to 3 cm off the midline, allowing for the overall shape of the muscle and variations in patient size, to ensure optimal assessment. The clinician may choose to firmly press the pad of their thumbs directly downward into the belly of each multifidus muscle or alternatively, begin a little more laterally then press downward and bring the thumbs slightly towards the midline. The clinician will determine which of these methods provides them with a more obvious appreciation for the differences in multifidus volume.

Frequently, at a specific level of the lumbar spine, the clinician will note a lack of multifidus symmetry between sides. The multifidus on one side may feel smaller, or less dense, as though it has lost some of its normal consistency when compared to the muscle above, below and contralateral to the involved segment. This test is very helpful for the clinician because, in conjunction with a thorough examination, it assists in the identification of the segmental level of pathology, and perhaps the side on which the bulk of the pathology exists in many patients. The extent to which the multifidus appears asymmetrical may also be useful from a prognostic perspective. If the opportunity presents itself, this clinical finding should be validated through more objective means such as ultrasound (US) or magnetic resonance imaging (MRI). Hides and colleagues demonstrated a high correlation between manual therapy assessment and US imaging in determining both the segment and the side at which multifidus volume had been lost (Hides et al., 1994).

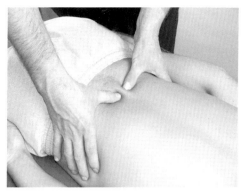

Figure 5.28 Palpation of lumbar multifidus muscle bulk.

Assessment of the Patient's Potential to Activate Transversus Abdominis

IN THEIR TEXT *Physiotherapy in Disorders of the Brain*, Carr and Shepherd describe motor skill as an expression of neuromuscular efficiency (Carr & Shepherd, 1980). They state that highly developed motor patterns occur without the recruitment of muscles which are inappropriate to the task. Thus learning or re-learning a new motor skill could be considered to be largely a process of shedding unnecessary muscle activations. Similarly, a person's motor skill potential depends on the extent to which they can minimize excessive or redundant activations.

The treatment plan for virtually all lumbar spine patients includes therapeutic exercises which require the patient to voluntarily and independently activate the transversus abdominis and multifidus. To a significant extent, their rehabilitative success depends on their ability to accurately perform these new patterns of muscular activation. Therefore, it is helpful from both a prognostic and a treatment planning perspective, to develop a rudimentary estimation of the case with which a given patient might learn these exercises.

This clinical test should be approached with the understanding that no one, regardless of the healthiness of their lumbar spine, has any inherent ability to voluntarily activate their transversus abdominis or their multifidus in isolation. This is not a 'can they or can't they' type of test. Rather, this simple clinical test provides the clinician with an appreciation for the number of substitution patterns which are initiated by the patient, an estimate of the amount of time required to teach the patient these exercises, the frequency with which the patient will need follow-up, the extent to which the patient will likely be dependent on external sources of feedback, and the patient's ultimate ability to perform the exercises with a high degree of precision.

With the patient in supine crook lying, the clinician uses their thumbs to palpate the lower abdominal wall, just medial and inferior to the anterior superior iliac spine (ASIS) (figure 5.29). The clinician's thumbs are thus in a position to palpate muscular activity in the lower abdominal wall, primarily in the internal oblique and the transversus abdominis muscles. A thumb position which is too close to the midline will result in palpation of rectus abdominis contraction rather than internal oblique and transversus abdominis. The clinician's fingers come to rest over the patient's posterolateral pelvis. This allows the clinician to palpate for contraction in muscles such as gluteus medius and gluteus maximus. The thenar eminence may also lay over the tensor fascia latae (TFL), which allows for monitoring of this muscle as well.

The clinician asks the patient to create a gentle tensioning in the lower abdomen directly under the clinician's thumbs. The patient is instructed to try to develop a subtle activation of the deep abdominals, maintain a relaxed breathing pattern and avoid the contraction of other trunk muscles. The clinician should *observe* the patient for evidence of contraction of muscles such the rectus abdominis (tensioning or bulging of the abdomen) the external oblique (depression of the rib cage),

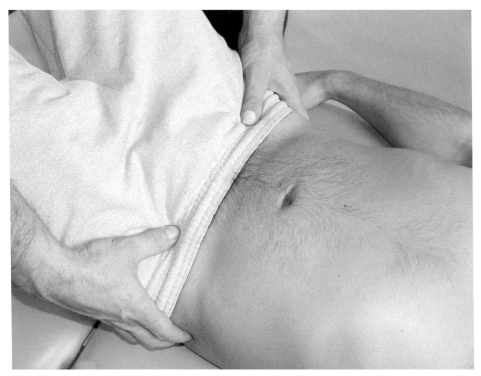

Figure 5.29 Palpation of the lower abdominal wall as the patient is asked to differentially activate their transversus abdominis muscle.

the hip flexors and adductors, the hamstrings and the superficial cervical flexors. Observation of the patient's breathing pattern also provides information as to their ability to dissociate their diaphragm from this attempted transversus abdominis activation. The patient should be monitored for any sign of lumbopelvic movement, into either a posterior or an anterior tilt.

An alternative approach is to ask the patient to gently contract their pelvic floor as if to prevent urination. Activation of the pelvic floor muscles facilitates activity in transversus abdominis (Sapsford et al., 2001; Neumann & Gill, 2002; Critchley, 2002). As this item is a part of the assessment (and not yet a component of the treatment plan) it is not necessary at this point to teach the patient everything they need to know about the pelvic floor and a correct pelvic floor contraction. However, if the patient is already familiar with pelvic floor exercises, the clinician can be somewhat more time efficient by having the patient utilize this approach. Once the patient has developed a more direct awareness of their transversus abdominis activation, the use of the pelvic floor contraction as a voluntary facilitating mechanism may be discontinued.

Regardless of whether the clinician asks the patient to gently activate the deep, lower abdominals or to gently contract their pelvic floor, an independent transversus abdominis activation is palpable as a subtle firming or tensioning of the lower abdominal wall. There is no sense of the internal oblique expanding or bulging into the clinician's thumbs. The patient continues to breathe in an appropriate and quiet manner and there is no evidence of other muscles being recruited. There is no sign of movement anywhere in the body. It is not unusual for the contraction of the transversus abdominis to be asymmetrical in patients with lumbar dysfunction. Symmetry of transversus abdominis activation should be monitored as the muscle must be active bilaterally in order to impact on segmental stiffness (Hodges et al, 2003). Any such asymmetry can also have serious effects on both the clinician's and the patient's perspective of how well the exercise is being performed. For example, the clinician may be pal-pating the side which is more active while the patient palpates the side with reduced activation.

Recall that at this point, we are not concerned with teaching the patient to correctly activate transversus abdominis; we are only interested in gaining a general appreciation of their skill level in terms of the performance of subtle motor activities. As per Carr and Shepherd's approach to motor re-learning, we are more interested in the degree to which the patient *can inhibit other muscles* and thus maintain an independent activation of transversus abdominis. The person with a higher degree of motor skill will demonstrate fewer co-contractions.

Conversely, the patient who clenches their teeth, forcefully recruits multiple muscles, holds their breath and moves into a posterior pelvic tilt when asked to gently contract only their deepest lower abdominal muscles will likely experience more difficulty learning to appropriately activate their transversus abdominis and multifidus as part of their therapeutic exercise program. Interestingly, the patient who fails on initial assessment to activate transversus abdominis, but manages to avoid contracting other muscles, will likely learn to activate transversus abdominis and multifidus much more quickly and with less need for interaction with the clinician.

A similar assessment process could be used with the multifidus; however, learning the multifidus activation is consistently more difficult for patients. Therefore, the patient's relative skill at activating transversus abdominis may be used as a general indicator of how difficult it will be for them to activate the segmental muscles.

Neurodynamic Testing

WHILE CLINICIANS ARE routinely aware of the need to test the mechanical behaviour of a patient's articular and muscular systems, the relevance of testing the mechanical behavior of the nervous system may not be as well appreciated. Neurodynamic testing provides a means of determining whether the connective and/or conductive tissues of the nervous system are able to tolerate mechanical loading similar to that experienced during physiological movement. Such testing is designed to provide information regarding the extent to which the neural tissues are involved in the patient's presentation. While there is limited evidence regarding the validity of neurodynamic testing, initial research appears promising (Coppieters et al, 2005).

As described previously, a restriction of the segment's tri-planar motion may develop secondary to a clinical instability if the neural control subsystem facilitates excessive activity in the multi-segmental muscles, altering the segment's normal axis of rotation. It has been hypothesized that if the nervous tissue itself is placed under excessive mechanical tension secondary to such an instability, the resulting neural irritability may trigger increased activity in these muscles as a means of reducing or limiting this tensioning. Clinically, this is evidenced by a decrease in segmental motion (in a segment determined to be dysfunctional during the course of assessment) which develops as the nervous tissue in the lower quadrant is placed under tension.

Each test should be explained to the patient in such a way that they feel free to report any sensation that arises during testing. They must be aware that *any* experience of pain or abnormal sensation must be reported to the clinician immediately to ensure safe application of the tests. The clinician must remember to standardize the test positions for each patient so as to optimize the reliability of the tests on subsequent testing. The patient's responses to neurodynamic testing may be interpreted as follows:

Physiological Response

The patient possesses a full, symmetrical and symptom free range of motion with the test. They may describe a mild to moderate pulling sensation but nothing which resembles their symptoms.

Clinical Response

The patient does not experience any degree of symptom reproduction in either the lumbar region nor the lower extremity during testing however there is an asymmetry in ROM between sides.

Neurogenic Response

There is both a reduction in ROM between the symptomatic and normal sides and a reproduction of the patient's symptoms. The patient's primary complaint of lumbar pain, neurogenic symptoms (paresthesia, dysesthesia or anesthesia) or lumbar pain along with neurogenic symptoms in the lower quadrant is reproduced. This response must be present before the nervous system can be implicated as being a source of the patient's symptomatic presentation. Sensitizing modifications can be applied to each test to provide further confirmation of the existence of a neurogenic component in the patient's presentation.

Typically, patients with clinical instabilities will present with some degree of altered neuro-dynamics. It is hypothesized that these changes are mediated by either chemical (inflammatory) or mechanical mechanisms related to the segmental dysfunction. It is essential for the clinician to appreciate that these neurodynamic deficits will frequently resolve as the clinical instability is corrected. That is, in most circumstances it does not appear necessary to direct any specific therapeutic intervention towards the neurodynamic deficits. In some cases, gentle therapeutic mechanical movement of neural tissues is indicated; these techniques are discussed further in chapter six.

The most commonly used neurodynamic tests in the lower quadrant are the Straight Leg Raise test (SLR), the Slump Test (ST) and the Femoral Nerve Tension Test (FNTT).

The Straight Leg Raise Test

This test is one of the more commonly utilized tests to assess neurodynamics in the lower quadrant. It is ideally suited to test the L4 - S1 nerve roots as well as the peripheral nerves to which they contribute, the sciatic, common fibular (peroneal) and the tibial nerves.

Complete patient comfort is important during this test so that a truly passive movement may be obtained. The patient is supine with their head supported on a pillow. The clinician is positioned on the side to be tested. The patient's knee is maintained in extension by the clinician's forearm. The clinician's other hand slowly elevates the lower limb *via* passive flexion of the hip (figure 5.30). Throughout range, the clinician evaluates the amount of connective tissue tension being developed. The clinician integrates this information with the point in the range of motion at which the patient reports any painful or abnormal sensation.

With the traditional SLR test, passive hip flexion is stopped at the point where the patient first experiences symptoms in the lower quadrant. The hip is then carefully extended to the point where these symptoms settle; the ankle is passively dorsiflexed. If the symptoms initially experienced with passive hip flexion are reproduced with dorsiflexion, the test is considered to have elicited a clinical or a neurogenic response depending upon the type of symptoms reproduced.

There are a variety of 'sensitizing' modifications which may be made to the traditional SLR test to provide additional information regarding the status of specific peripheral nerves in the lower limb (figures 5.31 - 5.33). This will be particularly helpful in determining the degree of neural tissue involvement in common patterns of lumbar dysfunction which can mimic the symptomatic presentations of conditions such as plantar fasciitis, ITB friction syndrome and trochanteric bursitis.

When utilizing these variations on the traditional SLR to assess patients with lower extremity symptoms (e.g., foot pain, lateral knee pain, lateral flank pain) it is important to add the sensitizing modification *prior* to raising the lower

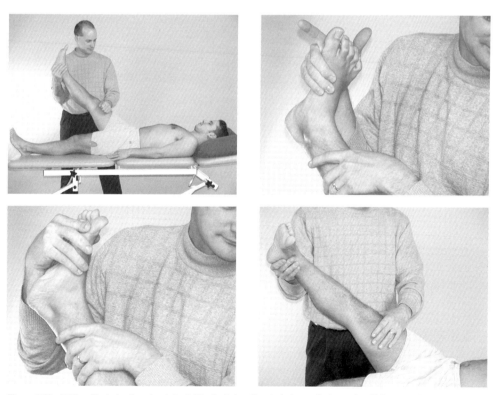

Figure 5.30 - 5.33 Clockwise from top left: **5.30** - Basic handling technique with the supine SLR test. **5.31** - SLR test plus dorsiflexion and eversion biases the test toward the tibial and medial plantar nerves. **5.32** - SLR test plus dorsiflexion and inversion biases the test toward the common fibular (peroneal) nerve. **5.33** - SLR test plus hip adduction and internal rotation biases the test toward the sciatic nerve.

extremity off the table. A good rule of thumb is to utilize the sensitizing modification which biases the test towards the component of the nervous system which the clinician wishes to evaluate. For example, when assessing a patient with 'plantar fasciitis', applying dorsiflexion and eversion first and then bringing the knee into extension and the hip into flexion biases the test more strongly to the medial plantar nerve which is believed to be involved in certain presentations of ongoing heel pain. The clinician may also ask the patient to flex and extend the cervical spine in an attempt to modify symptoms during any of these tests. This may provide further information regarding the effects of nervous tissue tension on the patient's symptoms.

The Slump Test

The Slump Test, a modification of the seated straight leg raise test, is not only useful for patients with lumbar and lower quadrant symptoms, but for also those with thoracic and cervical symptoms. The intention of the test is to sequentially tension the entire nervous system, including the lower brainstem, spinal cord, lumbar nerve roots and peripheral nerves of the lower quadrant.

 The patient sits at the side of the plinth with their arms either behind their back or resting lightly in their lap. The clinician is seated beside them to guide proper movement during the test and to assess for any changes in muscle tension through the trunk (figure 5.34). The patient is then asked to flex their thoracic and lumbar spine fully, followed by flexion of the cervical spine. From this flexed posture the patient actively extends one knee until they reach full extension or report any symptoms in the lower quadrant (figure 5.35). If the patient is able to fully extend the knee without reproducing their symptoms, one or both of the following sensitizing modifications may be added.

 The Slump Test plus dorsiflexion (figure 5.36) creates greater tensioning through the nervous system 'from below', while the Slump Test plus cervical extension reduces tension in the system 'from above'. The clinician may note the effect, if any, of these modifications on the patient's symptoms.

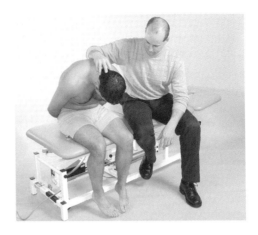

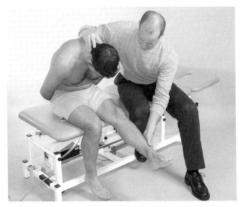

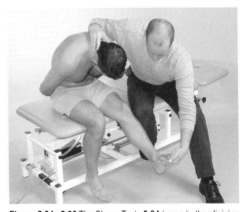

Figure 5.34 - 5.36 The Slump Test. **5.34** (upper) - the clinician guides the patient into the initial position of lumbar, thoracic and cervical flexion. **5.35** (middle) - guided by the clinician, the patient actively extends their knee to the point of either full extension or the onset of symptoms. **5.36** (lower) - if desired, the clinician may ask the patient to actively dorsiflex their ankle to determine if the patient's symptoms may be modified *via* this additional tensioning. Conversely, cervical extension may be added to determine if this 'de-tensioning' diminishes the patient's symptoms.

SCTs may be applied to the various segments of the lumbar spine while the patient is in the Slump Test position. The patient is positioned in a posture of neural tension just short of the point in range where initial pain is felt (i.e., P1). It is in this position that the SCT or a combined SCT may be applied to the segment of interest (figure 5.37).

The clinician must be aware of any increase in symptoms which result from the addition of these sensitizing movements. Furthermore, the clinician should note any differences in compliance when an SCT is performed with the spine in a position of neural tension relative to a non-tensioned posture. Either of these potential findings implicates the neural tissues as a component of the patient's presenting symptoms and provides additional information regarding the irritability of the condition. Alternatively, the Slump Test may be performed in side-lying; again, SCTs may be used to further investigate the effect of passive segmental motion on the patient's neural tension findings.

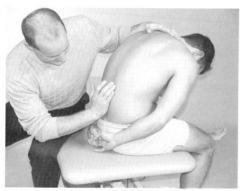

Figure 5.37 Segmental Compliance Testing in a position of increased neural tension. The clinician may choose to determine the effect of increased neural tension on segmental compliance at the dysfunctional segment. If so, the SCT should be tested at the point in range just prior to the onset of symptoms. The degree of connective tissue give with this test is then compared to that with the patient in sidelying.

Femoral Nerve Tension Test

This test is best utilized when one wishes to evaluate the nerve roots of the upper lumbar spine as well as the peripheral nerves to which they contribute. These include the femoral, ilioinguinal and saphenous nerves and as well as the lateral cutaneous nerve of the thigh.

The patient is positioned in side-lying with the side to be tested superior. They are placed in a fetal position with their hands holding their cervical spine into full flexion (figure 5.38). The clinician, using their more cranial hand, maintains the lumbopelvic region in a neutral posture and, and with their caudal hand, places the knee in as much flexion as possible. The hip is then brought into extension using the caudal hand (figure 5.39).

As the knee is passively flexed and the hip passively extended, the patient is asked to report any symptoms they are experiencing. As in the previous neurodynamic tests, the clinician makes note of where in range these symptoms appear and

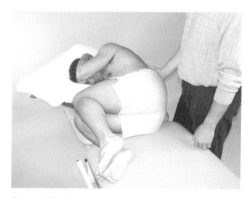

Figure 5.38 Femoral Nerve Tension Test - initial patient positioning. Patient is in a sidelying, fetal position with their cervical spine flexed and their lumbopelvic region maintained in a neutral posture.

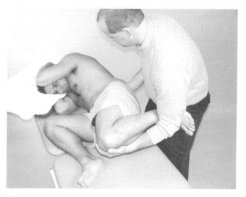

Figure 5.39 Femoral Nerve Tension Test - the clinician maintains the patient's neutral lumbopelvic posture and brings the superior knee into flexion and the hip into extension.

how this relates to the degree of connective tissue resistance noted through range.

The FNTT may be further sensitized by adding hip adduction which biases the test toward the lateral cutaneous nerve (figure 5.40). The clinician may also ask the patient to extend their cervical spine to assess the effect of decreased nervous system tensioning on the patient's symptoms and ROM (figure 5.41). Any effect on either the degree of tissue resistance as appreciated by the clinician or the patient's report of symptoms may provide the clinician with relevant information regarding the mechanical tolerances of the nervous system.

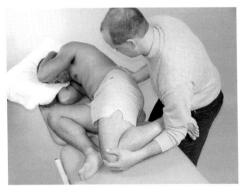

Figure 5.40 The Femoral Nerve Tension Test - the addition of passive hip adduction biases this test toward the lateral cutaneous nerve.

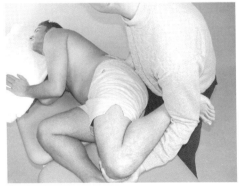

Figure 5.41 Once symptoms have been elicited *via* passive knee flexion, hip extension and potentially hip adduction, the clinician may ask the patient to extend their cervical spine so as to assess the effect of decreased nervous system tensioning on the patient's symptoms.

Neurological Screening Examination

THE PURPOSE OF A NEUROLOGICAL screening examination is to develop a basic appreciation for the state of the central and peripheral nervous systems in relation to the person with lower quadrant symptoms. This screening can help the clinician identify the patient who is not appropriate for physiotherapeutic intervention secondary to an undiagnosed central nervous system lesion and/or a progressive loss of peripheral nervous system function.

The neurological screening examination consists of assessment for the Babinski sign, clonus, lower quadrant reflexes, sensation and myotomal or 'key muscle' testing. The Babinski sign is assessed by running or dragging a firm thin object, such as the handle of a reflex hammer, along the lateral border of the foot and crossing over towards the base of the great toe (D1). The presence of the Babinski sign is indicated by a slow, involuntary combination of great toe extension and splaying of the remaining digits (the Babinski test is reported as either 'present' or 'absent', as opposed to the more typical 'positive' or 'negative'). The presence of the Babinski sign is indicative of a central nervous system lesion.

Clonus is most easily assessed by applying a rapid stretch to the ankle dorsiflexors and sustaining it without interruption. If there is a loss of descending motor inhibition, due to a central nervous system lesion, this stretch reflex continues unchecked, manifesting as an prolonged series of contractions of the ankle plantar flexors.

It should be noted that a CNS lesion is not necessarily a contraindication to physiotherapeutic intervention. People who have had previous CNS pathology frequently continue to demonstrate the presence of the Babinski sign and clonus. However, if a patient presents with previously undiagnosed CNS dysfunction, they must be referred back to their physician for further medical investigation and follow-up.

Table 5.1 Peripheral Nervous System Testing

Spinal Level	Myotome	Dermatome	Deep Tendon Reflex
L1	hip flexion	proximal anterior thigh	n/a
L2	hip flexion	proximal anterior thigh	n/a
L3	knee extension	distal anteromedial thigh	quadriceps
L4	ankle dorsiflexion	medial leg	quadriceps
L5	extension of D1	lateral leg, dorsum of foot	gastrocs, soleus
S1	plantar flexion	posterior leg and thigh	hamstrings, gastrocs

Myotome or Key Muscle Testing

When assessing myotomal function, consider not only the strength of the contraction but the rate at which the patient fatigues as the test is repeated. This fatigue may be due to simple disuse, or may indicate underlying neurological pathology. The patient with neurogenic weakness demonstrates a significant loss in muscle power after only three to five exertions. It is this rapid loss of muscle power, unassociated with pain, which is typical of neurogenic weakness. This differs from simple fatigue in that the loss of power is much more rapid in those with neurogenic weakness.

Clinicians should be watchful for the patient who demonstrates 'giving way' weakness with myotomal testing. This indicates either an inability or an unwillingness to sustain muscle power. Pain and pain avoidance are frequent causes of 'giving way' weakness.

Deep Tendon Reflex Testing

Reflex testing, as part of a neuromusculoskeletal examination, attempts to determine the presence or absence of the primary reflexes, as well as any hypo or hyperreflexia which may be present. Hyporeflexia, indicating a peripheral nervous system defect, and hyperreflexia, indicating CNS dysfunction, are not necessarily contraindicative for physiotherapy. However, the presence of altered reflexes must be reported to the patient's physician and monitored for signs of worsening.

Sensation

The assessment of sensation should include a variety of sensory inputs since each form of sensation takes a unique pathway along the CNS. It should also be kept in mind that, of the three forms of peripheral nervous system assessment, sensation testing is entirely subjective, while both myotomal and reflex testing are each more objective.

Other Factors Which May Modify a Patient's Prognosis

Multi-Level Segmental Dysfunction

Orthopaedic surgeons have found that operative techniques are generally more successful in patients with uni-level dysfunction. Likewise, conservative care clinicians should appreciate that the same is true for their interventions. The patient with a multi-level clinical instability has a much poorer prognosis than a patient with a similar degree of instability at a single segment. There is likely a limit to the extent to which our current conservative techniques can compensate for dysfunction in the passive, active and neural control subsystems.

Motor Control Skill

Another factor which may influence a patient's prognosis is the patient's general skill in terms of motor control. Although difficult to objectively assess in the clinical environment, clinicians are able to develop an *appreciation* for unusually low levels of motor skill in certain patients. Such patients may reasonably be expected to have a poorer prognosis given the motor skill requirements of this clinical model. Fortunately, only a very small percentage of patients are so motor-impaired as to render them incapable of learning to correctly activate their SSMs. The clinician's skill at education and facilitation of the SSMs is far more important. As the clinician becomes more proficient at teaching and assisting patients in developing voluntary control of the SSMs (an 'art' in the midst of much science), they note that fewer and fewer patients are 'unable' to learn these exercises.

Obesity

The clinical model described requires that the clinician be able to palpate activity in the transversus abdominis and lumbar multifidus muscles. If a patient is morbidly obese such that it is impossible to palpate these muscles, the clinician's ability to assess and facilitate this critical component of the program will be dramatically impaired. If the clinician has access to diagnostic ultrasound imaging for use as a form of biofeedback, this problem may be overcome (see page 129 for a discussion of diagnostic ultrasound as a biofeedback tool).

Psycho-Emotional Status

The patient's psycho-emotional status can affect the function of the neural control subsystem within the context of lumbar dysfunction. This is a broad category and may include any of the following:

- fear behaviours
- an inappropriately high self-impression of disability
- a tendency towards catastrophization
- subtle and overt secondary gain issues

- negative stressors
- anxiety and depression

The extent to which psychosocial disorders affect the success of physiotherapeutic intervention is, in the authors' opinion, generally under-appreciated by neuromusculoskeletal clinicians. When a competent and comprehensive assessment has been conducted, if either of the patient's reported pain experience or their level of function is not consistent with the clinician's objective findings, it should be considered a possibility that the patient's psycho-emotional status is affecting their neuromusculoskeletal presentation to a significant extent. At the same time, clinicians must take care to avoid arriving at this conclusion too easily. The wise clinician regularly questions if there might be something they have missed or if there is something they might do differently from a treatment perspective before assuming that a patient's failure to improve is due solely to psychosocial issues.

It is extremely rare for a patient to present with symptoms secondary only to psychosocial pathology. More typically, there is at least a measure of neuromusculoskeletal dysfunction which must be managed by the clinician. It is important that we be ever mindful of basing our management decisions on the patient's objective, rather than subjective, findings.

Diagnosis and Prognosis

THE INFORMATION GATHERED throughout the assessment is used to develop two closely related constructs: the diagnosis and the prognosis. Traditionally, a diagnosis is expected to identify the structure at fault and the degree of dysfunction. The diagnosis serves as the basis for the development of an effective management plan. The prognosis is a prediction regarding the extent to which the person will recover, and is based partly upon their diagnosis and partly upon a variety of other factors specific to the individual.

While a clinician may perform the Lachmann

test to assess the status of the anterior cruciate ligament, they are in fact assessing a number of structures which contribute to the control of anterior translation of the tibia relative to the femur. The clinician is actually performing a single test of the knee's passive subsystem in the anterior direction. The result of this ligamentous stress test and other examination items enables the clinician to describe with some certainty the extent of the patient's knee dysfunction and thus their prognosis. In such a case has the clinician actually developed a diagnosis? Clinicians appreciate that until this patient is assessed *via* arthroscopy, any clinical examination is unable to fully and accurately describe the precise injury. However, the clinical examination of the knee will frequently provide the clinician with enough information to develop an effective management plan and a reasonable prognosis. Does the patient require consultation with a surgeon or other medical evaluation, or can

they be expected to do well with conservative care alone? If the patient is considered non-surgical, what is the likelihood that they will return to full function and be fully symptom-free? Is the patient in need of enhanced dynamic stability, improved range of motion or both?

The segmental dysfunction model describes an approach to the clinical management of patients with lumbar dysfunction which is consistent with that considered appropriate in peripheral populations. The clinical spinal assessment described in this chapter enables the clinician to identify the location and the extent of the patient's segmental dysfunction, the biomechanical factors which perpetuate this dysfunction and the degree of their functional deficit. Management of the patient is then based upon the need to either restore or control segmental motion just as it is in patients with peripheral pathology.

management of lumbar segmental dysfunction

The conservative management of vertebral column pathology need not be seen as unusually complicated nor mystifying. Indeed, it need not be any more complex than the management of patients with peripheral joint dysfunction. As with other regions of the body, if the clinician understands the underlying anatomy, biomechanics, neurophysiology and pathophysiology and performs a well conducted initial assessment of the neuromusculoskeletal system, an appropriate diagnosis, prognosis and management plan will become readily apparent. The clinician who lacks this information will often find patient management to be unpredictable, confusing and frequently frustrating.

In consideration of the current evidence regarding spinal pathology, appropriate physiotherapeutic lumbar intervention, in the majority of cases, may be approached as a matter of managing the patient's segmental dysfunction. Given the ubiquitousness of the impairments affecting the deep segmental muscles, therapeutic segmental stabilization exercises will be a key component of patient management in the majority of cases. These are described in detail later in this chapter. In addition to these exercises, mobilization or manipulation will be necessary in situations where the patient's symptomatic segment is either excessively stiff and/or lacks adequate segmental motion. Mobilization and manipulation are also appropriate in the situation where the dysfunction at the symptomatic segment appears perpetuated by a lack of motion at some nearby segment. These techniques are described beginning on page 107. A novel application of therapeutic indwelling electrical muscle stimulation is also described.

Management of the patient with symptoms secondary to lumbar pathology emphasizes correction of the articular and neuromuscular dysfunction identified on assessment. While pain is the primary reason most patients choose to consult with a physiotherapist, it is recognized that pain is a complex, multi-dimensional experience which might not always prove amenable to physiotherapeutic intervention. As such, the issue of pain management should be approached with a degree of humility; our understanding of the pain experience, while certainly improving, remains relatively poorly developed. As knowledge in the field of pain research evolves, it is becoming apparent that pain is a more complex construct than had been previously believed. Fortunately, recent research has led to the development of new clinical models of pain management (Butler, 2000; Moseley, 2002; Butler and Moseley, 2003; Moseley, 2003). Such models provide clinicians with new insights into the mechanisms of pain and new therapies with which to modify certain pain states.

In the authors' opinion, while some patients will have more pain than segmental dysfunction, most patients with low back or lower quadrant pain will be found, on assessment, to have a degree and pattern of segmental dysfunction in keeping with their pattern of symptoms. The clinician must be mindful of the need to direct treatment towards the cause of the patient's symptoms, rather than toward the symptoms alone. Both the clinician and patient must be aware that the objective of treatment, as described in this text, is not pain management but segmental dysfunction management. In the majority of clinical circumstances, the restoration of adequate segmental motion and stability will coincide with a resolution of, or at least a marked improvement in, the patient's pain.

Rationale For the Use of Selected Treatment Techniques

THE PHYSIOLOGICAL RANGE of segmental motion has been partitioned into neutral zone and elastic zone components (Panjabi, 1992b). As discussed in chapter three, segmental motion through the neutral zone is that which occurs relatively freely, against only minimal internal resistance from the passive subsystem. Maitland demonstrated a clinical appreciation for these concepts *via* the movement diagram (Hickling & Maitland, 1970). Developed as a clinical tool to chart changes in joint behavior, a typical movement diagram closely parallels the stress-strain curve which became the foundation of Panjabi's neutral zone hypothesis (figure 5.10, page 84). Given the correspondence between these models, certain clinical interpreta-

tions of the Panjabi model seem reasonable. These interpretations are based upon both experimental and clinical evidence; clinical experience necessarily 'filling in the objective evidence gaps' which still exist regarding spinal pathomechanics.

As discussed previously, in most clinical circumstances, a patient's symptom generating segment will exhibit a decrease in segmental stiffness (or an increase in segmental compliance) as a direct result of the pathology affecting the passive components of that segment. In such cases, appropriate management would involve the rehabilitation of their segmental stabilizing muscles. However, on physical examination patients may also be found to have one or more spinal segments which demonstrate markedly decreased segmental compliance or give; traditionally, such segments are described as hypomobile. Clinically, the hypomobility may be considered to be a motion segment which no longer has adequate neutral zone motion (Lee, 1999d). In many such cases, appropriate management entails both rehabilitation of the segmental stabilizing muscles along with restoration of adequate compliance *via* mobilization or manipulation.

The mechanism underlying this loss of neutral zone motion remains unknown. It has been suggested that a marked increase in the resting tone of the lumbar multi-segmental muscles may alter the normal axis of rotation at a pathological motion segment which would otherwise be classified as being hypermobile given the deficit affecting the passive elements (Meadows, 2001). While this increased tone may represent an attempt by the neural control subsystem to 'splint' or 'brace' the dysfunctional segment, the resulting change in the axis of rotation is such that normal neutral zone motion is prevented from occurring at the involved segment. Instead of neutral zone motion being controlled efficiently, such motion is overly limited at the dysfunctional segment.

With a loss of neutral zone motion, any movement of the involved segment must occur against an increase in segmental stiffness, otherwise described as an increase in the segment's internal resistance to motion. In general, two clinical patterns may emerge from such a situation. In the first, the hypomobile segment behaves as an independent form of dysfunction. It may or may not be a symptom generating segment. In the second, the hypomobile segment effectively facilitates increased motion at a nearby segment. Since movement at the hypomobile segment must occur against greater internal resistance, it becomes biomechanically more efficient for movement to occur at the adjacent segment, a 'path of least resistance' phenomenon. If the adjacent segment becomes hypermobile, the neural control sub-system may become incapable of controlling this increased motion resulting in a *clinical instability*. In such cases, the clinician should identify and treat both the instability and its neighbouring hypomobility. Therapeutic segmental stabilization exercises may not be able to adequately train the neural control and active subsystems to compensate for the hypermobility if the adjacent hypomobility persists, perpetuating the increased segmental motion at the unstable segment. Mobilization and/or manipulation of the hypomobility as well as segmental stabilization exercises are required in these cases to fully manage such patients.

Mobilization & Manipulation

THE ABILITY OF THE CLINICIAN to specifically restore segmental motion in the lumbar spine is a fundamental component of patient management. Two interventions *via* which the clinician can achieve this are spinal mobilization and manipulation. Spinal mobilization describes a low velocity, relatively large amplitude technique used to improve connective tissue compliance and restore segmental motion. Manipulation refers to a high velocity, low amplitude thrust technique, also utilized to improve compliance and restore segmental motion. While both techniques can be effective at improving segmental motion and compliance, manipulation has certain advantages over mobilization: it results in greater improvements in segmental motion in significantly less time; and,

it generates specific therapeutic neurophysiological effects that mobilization does not.

There are three primary effects of spinal manipulation. Manipulation has been shown to increase connective tissue compliance - a mechanical effect - in a joint which has produced an audible 'pop' or cavitation and to decrease tone in the erector spinae muscles - a neurophysiological effect (Herzog, 2000). Clinically, it is suspected that this comb-ination of improved connective tissue compliance and altered muscle tone restores NZ motion. Manipulation has also been shown to induce an analgesic effect *via* activation of descending inhibitory pain pathways (Wright, 2000). In a recent review of the literature regarding the efficacy of manipulation in low back pain, Bronfort and colleagues found sufficient evidence to recommend manipulation as a viable intervention in both acute and chronic low back pain (Bronfort et al, 2004).

There are numerous clinical presentations which may benefit from mobilization and/or manipulation. If, on examination, a lumbar motion segment demonstrates limited segmental motion along with decreased segmental compliance (or increased segmental stiffness) mobilization and/or manipulation may be indicated. These techniques are to be used judiciously to restore segmental motion and not with the overt intention of restoring the patient's active range of motion nor improving their pain.

In the presence of clinical instability, the patient will frequently present with decreases in active range of motion of the trunk and pain with spinal movements. In such cases, despite the limitation of active trunk movement, motion at the dysfunctional segment may be excessive and poorly controlled. If the clinician's examination identifies this combination of limited trunk movement overlying an increase in segmental motion, mobilization and/or manipulation of the unstable segment is contraindicated.

Our assertion that mobilization and/or manipulation not be prescribed for pain control is based on the concern that both the clinician and the patient might neglect to participate in other therapeutic interventions which have far greater capacity to lead to a correction of the underlying segmental dysfunction. It is the authors' opinion that ongoing or repeated use of manipulation solely for the purpose of pain control is an inappropriate application of the therapy as it may detract from the utilization of other interventions requiring time and attention from both the clinician and the patient. Ongoing manipulation as a means of pain control may also facilitate a dependent relationship between the patient and the clinician whereby the patient may come to believe they require manipulative care in order to maintain control of their symptoms. Such a dependent relationship is not in the best interest of our patients and all means should be employed to avoid the development of such situations.

It is essential that the clinician base their decision to use mobilization and/or manipulation on an objectively determined need to restore segmental motion (*via* restoration of more normal NZ motion) and connective tissue compliance. Once this has been achieved, the patient's active trunk motion will be greater and oftentimes more comfortable. The extent of these improvements will depend on the current level of function of their segmental stabilizing muscles. In almost all clinical circumstances, once an improvement in segmental motion has been achieved, the focus of treatment should shift towards restoration of more optimal function of the neural and active subsystems.

Technical Review of Mobilization and Manipulation of the Lumbar Spine: General Principles

WHEN CONSIDERING A PERIPHERAL JOINT such as the shoulder, clinicians are generally comfortable with the concept that there is a fundamental difference between passive physiological range of motion (PROM) techniques and mobilization techniques intended to improve 'articular' stiffness or compliance. They appreciate that while the two are related, techniques utilized to restore articular compliance are applied at the end of the available ROM; there is no real movement to appreciate. While there may be some motion to be felt as the 'end feel' is approached, the actual mobilization itself works only into the available compliance of the articulation's soft tissues.

Spinal assessment and treatment is no different. PIVMs give information regarding which segment is problematic and in which direction the segment is restricted in terms of physiological movement. However, SCTs provide information regarding the specific component of that physiological movement which is stiff (or less compliant than normal) and thus, the component which needs to be mobilized or manipulated.

Grading

Articular mobilization techniques are generally graded on a five point scale from grade 1 mobilizations to grade 5 manipulations. Typically, grade 1 and 2 techniques are used clinically to modulate pain. There is no tension applied to the connective tissues of the segment at these grades. In the opinion of the authors, grade 1 and 2 mobilizations are far less effective and efficient than are other approaches to pain management including education, rest, ice and compression. Grade 3 to 5 techniques are utilized to restore segmental motion. This text will discuss grade 3 to 5 techniques, performed with the segment at its end range of physiological motion.

The Pre-Manipulative Hold

The pre-manipulative hold is a safety technique used to help ensure that a patient will be tolerant of manipulative treatment. The clinician applies a slow and steady force to the segment, in the position chosen for manipulation and with the same magnitude of force to be used in the technique (Pettman, 2000). The patient must not experience any discomfort or increase in muscle tone with the application of the pre-manipulative hold. If the pre-manipulative hold elicits any symptoms or an increase in muscle tone, the manipulation is considered to be contraindicated.

Positioning

The information presented in the following sections regarding patient positioning is critical. The target segment must be placed at the end of its available movement such that all appreciable 'give' or compliance in its connective tissue system is taken up. The patient is positioned in some combination of flexion or extension, sidebending and rotation so as to maximize the compressive and tensile forces acting at segments adjacent to the target segment. It is believed that this combination of patient and motion segment positioning will allow for the majority of the mobilization or manipulative force to be focused at the target segment. This clinical hypothesis regarding the efficacy of specific positioning is provided with some validity in that such exact positioning seems necessary for the therapeutic technique to be effective.

While it is important that the target segment and the segments adjacent to the target segment be positioned optimally, it is also important for the clinician to appreciate that any position utilized for mobilization or manipulation must be achievable without an increase in the patient's symptoms. The patient must be completely comfortable and relaxed. The patient's position must allow the target segment to be essentially symptom free with, at most, only slight tenderness to palpation. If these conditions cannot be met, it is in the best interests of all concerned that the mobilization or manipulation not be performed.

Lever Arms

It is helpful for the clinician to understand that the lumbar spine is the most difficult region of the spine to mobilize or manipulate. While this region of the spine is the simplest from a biomechanical perspective, the levers of the trunk, pelvis and lower extremities make any form of mobilization technically difficult. Once the clinician has established their own unique and subtle modifications to the technical instructions below, they will develop a level of comfort with mobilizations and/or manipulations.

Specific Lumbar Mobilization & Manipulation Techniques

"Anyone can learn to manipulate. The skilled have learned when not to."
Jim Meadows, PT, FCAMT

The following are detailed instructions regarding the technical issues of mobilization and manipulation in the lumbar spine. In the application of these techniques, the clinician's body becomes the treatment tool. Since clinicians themselves vary in shape and size they must modify these techniques in order to safely and effectively perform the interventions with a clinical population. Furthermore, effective performance of these techniques requires that the clinician develop a new set of motor skills. For these reasons, it will take some time to develop a level of proficiency adequate for clinical success.

The authors expect that clinicians will utilize only those techniques which are within their legislated scope of practice and which can be performed safely and effectively.

Direct and Indirect Techniques

A 'DIRECT' TECHNIQUE IS ONE in which the mobilizing or manipulative force is applied to the side of the lumbar spine which is closest to the clinician. 'Indirect' techniques are those with which the mobilizing or manipulative force is applied to the side of the spine which is closest to the plinth. Techniques 1 and 2 are direct techniques and are best utilized when no other segment in the lumbar spine is *symptomatic in the direction of the movement which is to be restored.* If even one lumbar segment, other than the target segment, is symptomatic in the same direction as the movement which is to be restored at the target segment, an indirect technique must be used.

For example, if the L4-5 segment was symptomatic into extension and the clinician was attempting to restore extension at L2-3, the direct techniques (techniques 1 and 2, below) would be contraindicated. In these instances, it is best to make use of an *indirect* technique at the target segment (as in techniques 3 and 4, below). In the infrequent situation where both direct and indirect techniques increase a patient's symptoms, mobilization and/or manipulation is contraindicated.

Direct Techniques

1. Flexion - Sidebending Technique

To illustrate this direct technique, a mobilization or manipulation of the right side of the L4-5 motion segment into flexion and left sidebending is described.

Clinical Objective
Restoration of segmental motion at a segment determined to be limited into flexion and left sidebending.

Positioning the Patient:
The patient is positioned in left side-lying. The clinician palpates the target segment and *via*

passive hip flexion, positions the target segment in full available flexion. This flexed position of the target must be maintained. The patient's lower extremities are then offset to facilitate side bending and rotation of the pelvis during the technique (figure 6.1). The patient's spine *superior to and including the target segment* must be placed in a position of maximal flexion and left sidebending; the patient's left arm is drawn anteriorly and caudally by the clinician until movement is appreciated through the target segment (figure 6.2).

Clinician's Hand Placement
With the patient properly positioned, the clinician's right hand slips under the patient's right arm such that the clinician's right thumb fixes the L4 spinous process from the lateral side of the spinous process. The palmar or anterior aspect of the clinician's left forearm rests in the space between the iliac crest and the greater trochanter (figure 6.3).

Delivery of the Technique
The clinician fixes the L4 spinous process *via* their right thumb. A pre-manipulative hold is performed. Assuming an appropriately safe response to the pre-manipulative hold, the clinician then mobilizes or manipulates using a caudal and lateral force delivered through the pelvis (figure 6.4). This can be delivered in a graded fashion (grade 3 to 5, either mobilization or manipulation) or as part of a static hold. If manipulating, it is best to apply the high velocity low amplitude thrust at the end of the patient's expiration. This facilitates maximum relaxation of the patient allowing for greater ease of application of the intervention.

Of Interest ...
While rotation is certainly produced by this technique, all efforts should be made to minimize it. The clinician maximizes their control of rotation by positioning the patient in such a way as to take up as much connective tissue compliance or 'give' as possible. This is achieved by careful positioning of the patient according to the directions above. In addition, the mobilizing or manipulating force must emphasize the sidebending of the pelvis rather than the rotation.

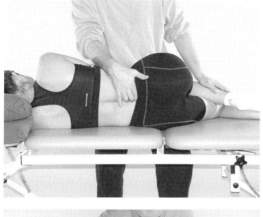 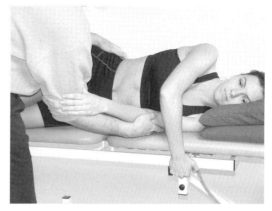

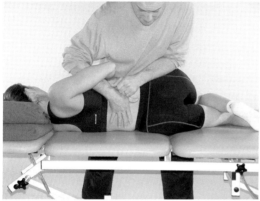 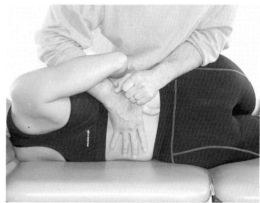

Figures 6.1 - 6.4 Direct Flexion - Left Sidebending Mobilization/Manipulation at L4-5. *Clockwise from upper left:* **Figure 6.1** - with the patient positioned in left side lying, the clinician palpates the target segment and positions this segment in full flexion. The patient's lower extremities are then off-set. **Figure 6.2** - the clinician draws the patient's left arm anteroinferiorly to position the target segment in maximum flexion and left sidebending. **Figure 6.3** - the clinician fixes the L4 spinous process from its lateral aspect and rests their other forearm in the space between the patient's iliac crest and greater trochanter. **Figure 6.4** - with the L4 vertebra fixed, the clinician mobilizes or manipulates the segment *via* a caudal and lateral force through the pelvis (if manipulating, a pre-manipulative hold is applied). The applied force must emphasize sidebending rather than rotation.

2. Extension & Sidebending Technique

To illustrate this direct technique, a mobilization or manipulation of the right side of the L2-3 motion segment into extension and right sidebending is described.

Clinical Objective
Restoration of segmental motion at a segment determined to be limited into extension and right sidebending.

Positioning the Patient:
The patient is positioned in left side-lying. The clinician palpates the target segment and, with the patient's knees fully flexed, passively extends the hips until the target segment is fully extended. This position must be maintained. The patient's lower extremities are then offset to facilitate side bending and rotation of the pelvis (figure 6.5). The patient's spine *superior to and including the target segment* must be placed in a position of maximal extension and right sidebending; to attain this posture, the patient's left arm is drawn anteriorly and cranially by the clinician (figure 6.6).

Clinician's Hand Placement
With the patient positioned properly, the clinician's right hand slips under the patient's right arm such that the clinician's right thumb fixes the L2 verte-

112

bra from the lateral aspect of its spinous process. The palmar aspect of the clinician's left forearm rests in the space between the iliac crest and the greater trochanter (figure 6.7).

Delivery of the Technique

The clinician fixes the L2 spinous process *via* the right thumb. A pre-manipulative hold is performed. Assuming an appropriately safe response to the pre-manipulative hold, the clinician then mobilizes or manipulates using a cranial and medial force delivered through the pelvis (figure 6.8). This can be delivered in a graded fashion (grade 3 to 5, either mobilization or manipulation) or as part of a static hold. If manipulating, it is best to apply the high velocity low amplitude thrust at the end of the patient's expiration. This facilitates maximum relaxation of the patient allowing for greater ease of application of the manipulative thrust.

Of Interest ...

While rotation is certainly produced with this technique, all efforts should be made to minimize it. The clinician maximizes their control of rotation by positioning the patient in such a way as to take up as much connective tissue 'give' as possible. This is achieved by careful positioning of the patient according to the directions above. In addition, the mobilizing or manipulating force must emphasize the sidebending of the pelvis rather than the rotation.

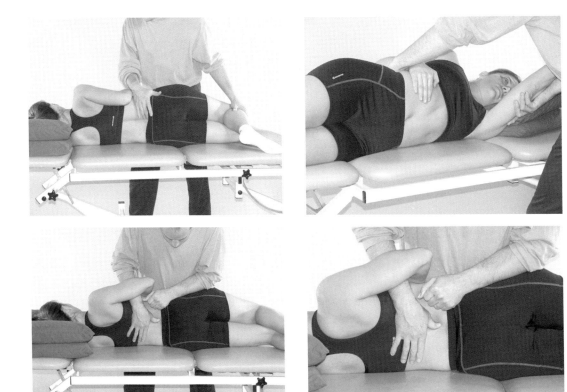

Figures 6.5 - 6.8 Direct Extension - Right Sidebending Mobilization/Manipulation at L2-3. *Clockwise from upper left:* **Figure 6.5** - with the patient positioned in left side-lying, the clinician palpates the target segment and positions this segment in full extension. The patient's lower extremities are then off-set. **Figure 6.6** - the clinician draws the patient's left arm anterosuperiorly to position the target segment in maximum extension and right sidebending. **Figure 6.7** - the clinician fixes the L2 spinous process from its lateral aspect and rests their other forearm in the space between the patient's iliac crest and greater trochanter. **Figure 6.8** - with the L2 vertebra fixed, the clinician mobilizes or manipulates the segment *via* a cranial and medial force through the pelvis (if manipulating, a pre-manipulative hold is applied). The applied force must emphasize sidebending rather than rotation.

Indirect Techniques

3. Flexion & Sidebending Technique

To illustrate this indirect technique, a mobilization or manipulation of the right side of the L4-5 motion segment into flexion and left sidebending is described.

Clinical Objective
Restoration of segmental flexion and sidebending in the lumbar spine when flexion above or below the target segment is painful.

Positioning the Patient
The patient is positioned in right side-lying. The clinician palpates the target segment and *via* passive hip flexion, positions the target segment in full available flexion. This flexed position of the target must be maintained. The patient's lower extremities are then offset to facilitate side bending and rotation of the pelvis (figure 6.9). The patient's spine *superior to and including the target segment* must be placed in a position of maximal flexion and left sidebending; the patient's right arm is drawn anteriorly and cranially by the clinician until this positioning is attained (figure 6.10).

Clinician's Hand Placement
With the patient positioned properly, the clinician's left hand slips under the patient's left arm, such that the clinician's left thumb fixes the L4 spinous process from the lateral side of the spinous process. The palmar aspect of the clinician's right forearm rests in the space between the iliac crest and the greater trochanter (figure 6.11 - next page).

Delivery of the Technique
The clinician fixes the L4 spinous process *via* the left thumb. A pre-manipulative hold is performed. Assuming an appropriately safe response to the pre-manipulative hold, the clinician then mobilizes or manipulates using a cranial and medial force delivered through the pelvis (figure 6.12 - next page). This can be delivered as a graded technique (grade 3 to 5, either mobilization and manipulation) or as part of a static hold. If manipulating, it is best to apply the high velocity, low amplitude thrust at the end of the patient's expiration. This facilitates maximum relaxation of the patient allowing for easier application of the technique.

Of Interest ...
While rotation is certainly produced with this technique, all efforts should be made to minimize it. The clinician maximizes their control of rotation

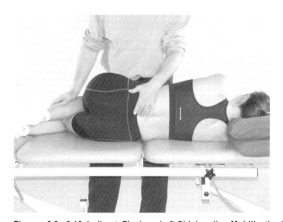
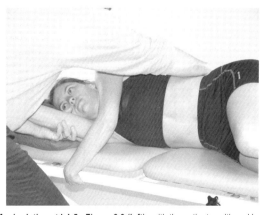

Figures 6.9 - 6.10 Indirect Flexion - Left Sidebending Mobilization/Manipulation at L4-5. Figure 6.9 (left) - with the patient positioned in right side-lying, the clinician palpates the target segment and positions this segment in full flexion. The patient's lower extremities are then offset. **Figure 6.10 (right)** - the clinician draws the patient's right arm anterosuperiorly to position the target segment in maximum flexion and left sidebending.

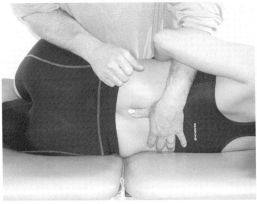 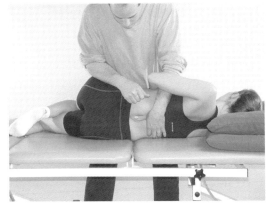

Figures 6.11 - 6.12 Indirect Flexion - Left Sidebending Mobilization/Manipulation at L4-5. **Figure 6.11 (left)** - the clinician fixes the L4 spinous process from its lateral aspect and rests their other forearm in the space between the patient's iliac crest and greater trochanter. **Figure 6.12 (right)** - with the L4 vertebra fixed, the clinician mobilizes or manipulates the segment *via* a cranial and medial force through the pelvis (if manipulating, a pre-manipulative hold is applied). The applied force must emphasize sidebending rather than rotation.

by positioning the patient in such a way as to take up as much connective tissue 'give' as possible. This is achieved by careful positioning of the patient according to the directions above. In addition, the mobilizing or manipulating force must emphasize the sidebending of the pelvis rather than the rotation.

4. Extension & Sidebending Technique

To illustrate this indirect technique, a mobilization or manipulation of the right side of the L2-3 motion segment into extension and right sidebending is described.

Clinical Objective
Restoration of segmental extension and sidebending in the lumbar spine when extension above or below the target segment is painful.

Positioning the Patient
The patient is positioned in right side-lying. The clinician palpates the target segment and, with the patient's knees fully flexed, passively extends the hips until the target segment is positioned in full extension. This extended position of the target must be maintained. The patient's lower extremities are then offset to facilitate side bending and rotation of the pelvis (figure 6.13).

The patient's spine *superior to and including the target segment* must be placed in a position of maximal extension and right sidebending; the patient's left arm is drawn anteriorly and caudally by the clinician until this positioning is achieved (figure 6.14).

Clinician's Hand Placement
With the patient properly positioned, the palmar aspect of the clinician's left hand slips under the patient's left arm such that the clinician's left thumb may fix the L2 vertebrae from the lateral aspect of the spinous process (figure 6.15). The palmar aspect of the clinician's right forearm rests in the space between the iliac crest and the greater trochanter.

Delivery of the Technique
The clinician fixes the L2 spinous process with their left thumb. A pre-manipulative hold is performed. Assuming an appropriately safe response to the pre-manipulative hold, the clinician asks the patient to fully relax and the clinician then mobilizes or manipulates using a caudal and lateral force delivered through the pelvis (figure 6.16). This can be delivered in a graded fashion (grade 3 to 5, either a mobilization or a manipulation) or as part of a static hold. If manipulating it is best to apply the high velocity low amplitude thrust at the end of the patient's expiration. This facilitates maximum relaxation of the patient allowing for greater ease of application of the manipulative thrust.

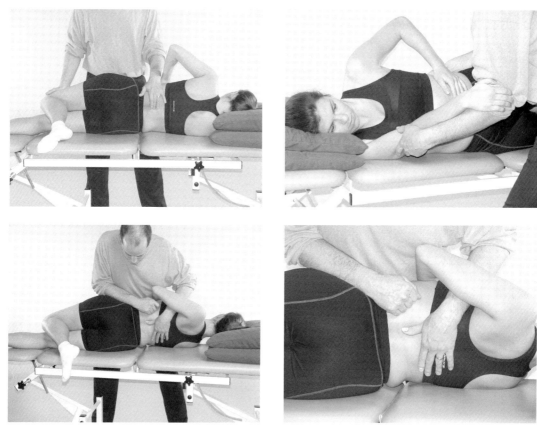

Figures 6.13 - 6.16 Indirect Extension - Right Sidebending Mobilization/Manipulation at L2-3. *Clockwise from upper left:* **Figure 6.13** - with the patient positioned in right side lying, the clinician palpates the target segment and positions this segment in full extension. The patient's lower extremities are then off-set. **Figure 6.14** - the clinician draws the patient's right arm anteroinferiorly to position the target segment in maximum extension and right sidebending. **Figure 6.15** - the clinician fixes the L2 spinous process from its lateral aspect and rests their other forearm in the space between the patient's iliac crest and greater trochanter. **Figure 6.16** - with the L2 vertebra fixed, the clinician mobilizes or manipulates the segment *via* a caudal and lateral force through the pelvis (if manipulating, a pre-manipulative hold is applied). The applied force must emphasize sidebending rather than rotation.

Of Interest ...

While rotation is certainly produced with this technique, all efforts should be made to minimize it. The clinician maximizes their control of rotation by positioning the patient in such a way as to take up as much connective tissue 'give' as possible. This is achieved by careful positioning of the patient according to the directions above. In addition, the mobilizing or manipulating force must emphasize the sidebending of the pelvis rather than the rotation.

Any of the preceding mobilization and/or manipulation techniques can be performed repeatedly over the course of treatment. It must be remembered that these techniques are utilized only until segmental motion is restored and then maintained by an improvement in the activation and control of the segmental stabilizing muscles.

Rehabilitation of the Segmental Stabilizing Muscles

In Chapter 5, a clinical test used to gain a general appreciation of the patient's potential to activate their transversus abdominis is described. In this section, therapeutic rehabilitation of the transversus abdominis and multifidus muscles is discussed in detail.

A variety of muscles in the lumbar region may contribute to the control of lumbar segmental motion. The multi-segmental paraspinal and abdominal muscles, *via* heightened activation and co-contractive patterning, are capable of both controlling segmental motion and maintaining the general orientation of the spine. However, there are problems associated with the use of these muscles for the purpose of segmental motion control. Increased loading of the spinal tissues (Marras et al, 2001; Ferguson et al, 2004), excessive restriction of segmental motion (Lee, 1999d; Meadows, 2001), restriction of the mobility of peripheral nervous tissues (Butler, 2000) and impairments in respiratory function (Hodges & Moseley, 2003; Hodges, 2004) have all been described as being either actual or potential negative outcomes associated with this strategy. Additionally, although the neural control subsystem appears to utilize the multi-segmental muscles for the purpose of achieving spinal stability in patients with low back pain (van Dieen et al, 2003a), the high incidence of recurrent and chronic back pain suggests that this strategy is not especially effective.

The deep segmental muscles are considered to be architecturally suited to the control of tri-planar segmental motion (Jemmett et al, 2004), and in such a way as to maintain optimal segmental mobility without excessive spinal rigidity nor the various deleterious sequelae described above (Hodges, 2004). Biomechanical studies have demonstrated the potential for these muscles to generate intersegmental stiffness (Panjabi et al, 1989; Kaigle et al, 1995; Quint et al, 1998; Hodges et al, 2003). Further, neurophysiological studies support the contention that the neural control subsystem utilizes the deep segmental muscles for the purposes of segmental motion control in non-pathologic populations (Hodges & Richardson, 1996; Moseley et al, 2002). Thus, under normal circumstances, it appears that muscles such as the transversus abdominis and deep multifidus are employed to generate intersegmental stiffness and control segmental motion. However, the deep segmental muscles have been shown to experience a variety of deficits in association with low back pain. Specific histochemical, morphological, and electrophysiological changes have been reported in patients with low back pain, with these changes occurring in the transversus abdominis, multifidus and psoas muscles. A comprehensive review of this literature is provided in chapter three, page 42. Given this literature, the objective of our therapeutic exercises in the management of patients with lumbar dysfunction should be to improve the function of the deep segmental muscles such that they might generate sufficient intersegmental stiffness to compensate for any underlying increase in NZ motion.

In the authors' opinion, muscle endurance training, pilates and yoga exercises, swimming, and stability ball exercises, while they may be performed 'gently', are each highly complex motor skills which place extraordinary motor control demands on the neural control subsystem. Indeed, they are likely so 'motor complex' that they will *overwhelm* the neural control sub-system's capacity to correctly activate muscles such as transversus abdominis and multifidus in patients with lumbar dysfunction. This may well explain why the aforementioned histochemical, morphological and neurophysiological changes persist in people with low back pain and why a variety of therapeutic exercise options, each of which involve anti-gravity, gross-motor skills, show only similar efficacy in terms of a degree of symptomatic improvement (Mannion et al, 1999). It is worth noting that such exercises have not been shown to reduce a patient's risk of future symptomatic episodes.

Finally, the traditional physiotherapeutic management of patients with low back pain typically includes exercises such as lumbar extension from a quadruped position or gentle 'abdominal exercises'; there is a significant body of research demonstrating that such interventions do little to positively impact upon the course of either acute or chronic low back pain (van den Hoogen et al, 1997; Frost et al, 2004).

A therapeutic exercise intervention based on motor re-education concepts, described originally for use in neurological rehabilitation (Carr & Shepherd, 1980), has been modified for use in lumbar populations (Richardson et al, 1999). Essentially, the model requires that patients learn to voluntarily activate, as independently as possible, their transversus abdominis and multifidus muscles. It is hypothesized that once the neural control subsystem can recruit these muscles independently of the other trunk muscles, normal patterns of activation may be restored resulting in increased intersegmental stiffness and improved control of NZ motion. Research published by the developers of this approach demonstrates that this clinical model can restore the pathological multifidus to a normal CSA within six weeks and, over a three year follow-up period, dramatically reduce the patient's risk of experiencing future low back pain episodes (Hides et al, 1996; Hides et al, 2001). Clinical outcomes studies of this model of therapeutic exercise in both acute and chronic populations have been published (Hides et al, 1996; O'Sullivan et al, 1997; Hides et al, 2001; Niemisto et al, 2003; Brox et al, 2003; Shaughnessy & Caulfield, 2004).

The therapeutic exercise intervention may be described as a five stage process:

1. Independent Activation

2. Tonic Hold

3. Integrated Tonic Hold

4. Dynamic Activation

5. Integrative Training

It should be noted that each of these five stages represents a skill set which must be attained by the patient. The intervention will break down if stages are skipped or a patient is permitted to only partially develop any skill level. The precise methods by which each of these skill sets are achieved varies somewhat from patient to patient and between clinicians. Different patients must overcome different challenges as they attempt to attain each skill. We suggest that clinicians develop a repertoire of modifications to their basic approach in order to meet the numerous coaching challenges posed by the different patients encountered in clinical practice. The skills developed during the fifth stage, Integrated Training, will vary and will be dependent upon the patient's activities of daily living including their occupational, recreational and sports activities.

In accordance with traditional motor re-education principles, the clinician may utilize a variety of environmental contexts and coaching techniques to enhance patient success. The initial teaching and rehearsal of these techniques is best conducted in a quiet room, away from noise and distraction. The clinician should adopt a nurturing, calm vocal style to lessen any anxiety the patient may feel as they attempt these difficult techniques. Instructions should be stated in clear, simple terms. The clinician should recognize that a given patient may be capable of attending only to a single component of a given skill (for example, minimizing contraction in the external oblique) during a single treatment session and that it may not be possible to achieve all components of a certain skill set in one day. A treatment session might conclude with the patient activating their transversus abdominis while having learned to minimize activity in external oblique, yet they continue to hold their breath; this can be the focus of the next treatment session. The clinician should also bear in mind that most patients will be limited to, at most, ten to fifteen minutes of focused exercise time, given the demands of such concentration-heavy exercises.

Stage One:
Independent Activation - Transversus Abdominis

The clinician must allow sufficient time to educate the patient regarding the rationale supporting this approach, their relevant trunk anatomy and the desired exercise technique. This is critical to gaining the patient's confidence and their compliance. If necessary, education alone might reasonably consume an entire treatment session. The clinician must also determine how far to take the patient during any single exercise session, how frequently they should be brought in for follow-up and which mode of feedback (tactile, verbal, visual, surface electromyography) will be most helpful for them at any given stage.

Readers may be familiar with certain verbal cues used to help patients learn to differentially activate the transversus abdominis. Cues such as 'draw your belly button into your spine', 'create a concave lower abdomen', or 'pull your belly away from the inside edge of your pant's waistband' have become common in clinical practice. Each of these cues implies that some motion of the abdominal wall should take place. Since the clinical effectiveness of this approach is in large part dependent upon the degree to which the patient can activate transversus abdominis **independently of the other trunk muscles**, the clinician must ensure that the patient activates transversus abdominis while minimizing activity in the remaining trunk muscles. In the authors' opinion, the above cues often lead to excessive contraction of the rectus abdominis, external oblique and/or internal oblique. Indeed, some patients will contract a number of trunk and lower extremity muscles when attempting to mobilize their abdominal wall.

The facilitation technique we recommend involves a gentle contraction of the anterior pelvic floor to facilitate activation of transversus abdominis. While a gentle pelvic floor contraction facilitates isolated activity in transversus abdominis (Sapsford et al, 2001), an aggressive or forceful pelvic floor contraction also recruits other abdominal muscles. The clinician must educate the patient in regard to their pelvic floor anatomy, various techniques of pelvic floor contraction and

the benefit of concentrating on their pelvic floor as opposed to their abdominal muscles. If at all possible, the patient should attempt to contract only the anterior half of the pelvic floor; clinically, this seems to minimize contraction of the gluteal muscles. The pelvic floor muscles may be described to patients in a variety of ways. They may be described as a 'relaxed hammock' strung between the tailbone and pubic bone. With female patients, the clinician may choose to simply say 'think of the pelvic floor as your vaginal muscles'.

In terms of contraction technique, both men and women often respond well to the analogy of bladder control. Indeed, asking a patient to initially practice this activation while urinating is sometimes helpful. The patient is instructed to stop their urine flow using the least amount of effort necessary in order to avoid a widespread contraction of their abdominal, hip and pelvic muscles. Using the relaxed hammock analogy, the patient may imagine trying to create tension in this hammock and gently draw it 'inside' their body (figure 6.17).

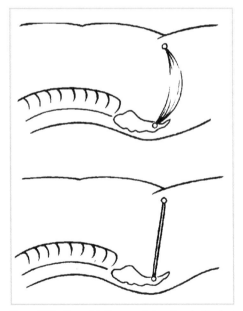

Figure 6.17 The pelvic floor as a 'relaxed' and a firm hammock. Certain patients will find this a useful visualization to help them activate their transversus abdominis *via* their pelvic floor. Asking the patient to focus on gently contracting the anterior portion of the 'hammock' seems to help minimize contraction of the gluteal muscles (from *Spinal Stabilization - The New Science of Back Pain, 2nd Ed.*, with permission).

With female patients, and specifically those who have previously performed *Kegel* exercises, simply reminding the patient of these exercises is usually sufficient. Men often find they can contract their pelvic floor if they imagine their testicles as sitting outside the body but at the open end of two hollow tunnels extending into the body. As they attempt to draw their testes back inside, a pelvic floor contraction is developed. To assist patients in developing a specific, gentle pelvic floor contraction (and thus our primary objective - the activation of the transversus abdominis muscle independent of the superficial abdominal muscles), it is often helpful to suggest that they think of this as a pelvic floor exercise instead of an abdominal exercise. With some patients, this helps minimize excessive contraction of the superficial abdominal wall.

It is most important to begin these exercises in a position of patient comfort. The patient may be positioned in either supine crook-lying, side-lying or prone-lying* and with their lumbar spine in a neutral lordosis. In supine there is no need to modify the patient's lordosis so long as they are comfortable; in prone a pillow placed under the abdomen is often necessary. Patient comfort should be the clinician's primary consideration in selecting the position in which to begin these exercises. Most patients will be most comfortable in supine crook-lying, thus the exercises are described using this as the patient's starting position.

With the patient in supine crook-lying, their head resting on a pillow, the clinician, using their thumbs, palpates the lower lateral abdomen bilaterally, just medial and inferior to the ASISs (figure 6.18). The clinician's fingers come to rest around the patient's posterolateral pelvis, able to palpate contraction of the gluteal muscles. The clinician observes the patient's neck, thoracic region, abdomen and hips for signs of co-contraction in the sternocleidomastoid (SCM) & scalenes, external oblique, diaphragm, rectus abdominis and hip adductors and flexors.

The clinician palpates the lower abdominal wall for activation of the internal oblique and transversus abdominis. Their thenar eminence may also be used to palpate for contraction in the tensor fascia latae (TFL) muscles. If the clinician suspects

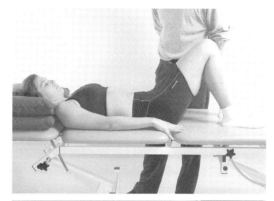

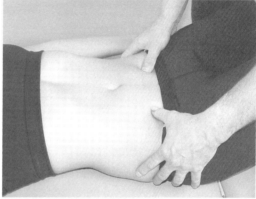

Figure 6.18 Supine crook-lying is frequently a comfortable position for patients with lumbar dysfunction and allows the clinician to readily palpate the lower abdominal wall, and observe for signs of compensatory muscle contractions. The clinician palpates the lower abdominal wall just medial and inferior to the patient's ASIS bilaterally.

that the hamstring or gluteal muscles are contracting, they may place the fingers of one hand under one of the patient's heels; if the patient is contracting their hamstring or gluteal muscles, the clinician will feel the heel compress into their fingers. Continue to monitor the lower abdominal wall using the other hand (figure 6.19).

The patient is asked to breathe in, exhale and gently contract their pelvic floor, while the clinician palpates and observes as described above. If the transversus abdominis activates independently, the clinician will appreciate a very subtle tensioning of the lower abdominal wall. There will be no sense of the lower abdominal wall rising or 'pushing out' into the clinician's thumbs (indicating internal oblique contraction), no movement of the ribcage indicative of external oblique contraction and the rectus abdominis remains quiet. The hips appear

* Patients frequently find their low back pain to be exacerbated with the prone posture; use this position with discretion.

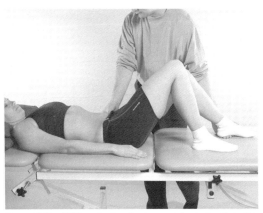

Figure 6.19 While palpating the lower abdominal wall on the patient's symptomatic side, the clinician may also palpate for a variety of unwanted, compensatory contractions. In this example, the clinician monitors for activation of the left side hip extensors in addition to the lower abdominal wall. If the patient contracts her hip extensors, her heel will press further into the clinician's fingers.

to remain relaxed and no additional contraction is noted in the gluteals or the TFL. The patient's superficial neck flexors appears relaxed and they can continue breathing normally.

Typically this ideal pattern is not developed on the patient's first attempt. Patients frequently hold their breath, contract all their abdominal muscles and move into a posterior pelvic tilt (probably because when the clinician *said* pelvic 'floor' the patient *heard* pelvic 'tilt'). The ribcage depresses as the external oblique contracts and the patient's attempt to contract their pelvic floor results in a mass action of the gluteal muscles. Correction of this involves application of the motor learning principles briefly described earlier. The clinician learns with time that patients often present with certain incorrect patterns containing several flaws, and that these may be corrected one flaw at a time across two, three or four treatment sessions. The clinician may take one of two general approaches. With the first, the initial emphasis is on the activation of transversus abdominis; so long as this occurs, other incorrect contractions are tolerated then dealt with one at a time. Alternatively, no incorrect contractions are permitted and the emphasis is on minimizing all flawed patterns while allowing the transversus abdominis activation to develop with time. In the authors' experience, the former is often more motivational for the patient, as they have at least achieved activity in the target muscle.

Frequently, the clinician notes that there is an asymmetrical activation of the transversus abdominis in patients with low back pain. Sometimes this asymmetry takes the form of a delayed, sluggish activation on one side and sometimes there is simply not the same degree of activity on one side. In either circumstance, this seems to improve with practice and without the patient necessarily needing to focus on correcting the asymmetry. Recent research has provided evidence that a unilateral activation of the transversus abdominis is not capable of controlling segmental motion (Hodges et al, 2003).

Patients often demonstrate improved activation within a single session as their clinician provides them with encouraging, appropriate cueing and sufficient time and opportunity to work out their 'glitches'. There are numerous examples from our practice where all a patient needed to develop this skill was some encouragement and practice time. In most cases, the clinician may find it best to avoid an ongoing critique of each attempt and simply allow the patient to learn through their own physical experience.

In reality there is no 'correct' method by which all patients are facilitated through any of these five stages. The only correct approach is the one which brings the patient to the desired goal. In the first stage, the goal is a voluntary, differential activation of transversus abdominis followed by the same of the multifidus. Whatever the clinician has to do to help the patient attain this objective is the 'right' thing to do in that specific situation.

Stage One
Independent Activation - Multifidus

Conceptually, this is identical to the initial activation of transversus abdominis. The objective is the learned skill of a voluntary, differential activation of multifidus at the dysfunctional segment. This is best taught in either supine crook or prone-lying. If the patient is in supine, the clinician simultaneously palpates both the transversus abdominis and multifidus on the same side. The bulk of the treatment time should be spent facilitating activity on the symptomatic side, and with regard to multifidus, specifically at the level of dysfunction. The dysfunctional segment and side will have been determined during the initial assessment. If the patient is in prone, the clinician will palpate the bilateral multifidus, again at the specific dysfunctional segment. Supine crook-lying is described first.

When the patient is comfortably positioned in supine crook-lying, the clinician stands on the patient's affected side facing the patient. The patient is asked to keep their back muscles very relaxed while the clinician places their more cranial hand under the patient, with their palm facing the patient's back. The clinician slides this hand under the patient so that the tip of their middle finger just reaches the L5 spinous process. From this starting position, the clinician locates the dysfunctional segment and presses the tip of the middle finger 'up' into the multifidus muscle adjacent to this target segment. The clinician should keep their finger very close to the midline so as not to mistake activity in longissimus for activity in multifidus. With the clinician's finger tip in multifidus, they can palpate the longissimus and iliocostalis using more palmar aspects of the same hand. The clinician's caudal hand (first two fingers) palpates the transversus abdominis on the same side (figure 6.20).

If the clinician is confident that the patient will tolerate several minutes of prone-lying without experiencing a significant increase in symptoms, the initial activation work for multifidus may be done in prone. A pillow is placed under the patient's abdomen and another pillow under their shins; the patient's head and neck are aligned comfortably in the *face-rest* of the plinth. The clinician locates the dysfunctional segment and places their thumbs gently but firmly into the adjacent right and left multifidus within a centimeter (the length of a thumb nail) of the spinous process (figure 6.21). This provides the patient with a 'target' at which to focus their efforts.

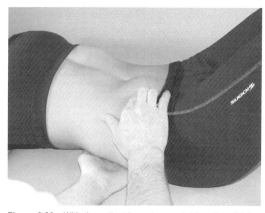

Figure 6.20 With the patient in supine crook-lying, the clinician may palpate both the lower abdominal wall and the lumbar musculature as the patient learns to differentially activate their multifidus muscle at the dysfunctional segment. The clinician's cranial hand palpates the multifidus at the dysfunctional segment using the tip of the middle finger. The more lateral lumbar musculature may also be palpated *via* this same hand.

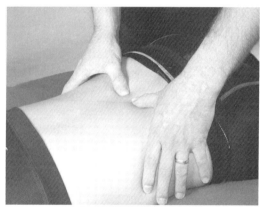

Figure 6.21 With the patient in prone lying, the clinician may palpate the lumbar multifidus bilaterally. The clinician's thumbs are used to appreciate the degree and quality of multifidus activation relative to more lateral trunk muscles.

With regard to verbal cueing for multifidus, clinicians have somewhat fewer options than for transversus abdominis. The patient can be asked to 'gently swell the muscle' into the clinician's finger. While this is a common cue, we have found it to be less than satisfactory; rarely does this seem to work as well as do other cues. Another cue involves the patient imagining that they are squeezing their multifidus towards the midline of the spine, without allowing any actual movement to occur. The clinician may teach this to patients by asking them to think of the feeling of squeezing their buttocks together; the patient then tries to have their multifidus do the same. Alternatively, the patient may be asked to *pretend* to gently arch or extend their lumbar spine without actually moving at all. The clinician should explain to the patient that these are imagined or 'virtual' movements, they happen only in the mind. These last two options have been found, in the authors' clinical experience, to be more consistent in helping patients activate the lumbar multifidus.

With the patient comfortably positioned and the clinician palpating the multifidus, the patient is asked to breathe in, exhale gently and activate their multifidus as per the selected cue. As they do so, the clinician palpates the multifidus and observes the patient for signs of co-contraction in other muscles. Common patterns of co-contraction include the external oblique, which can be noticed by movement of the lower anterolateral ribcage. Some patients create a general static contraction throughout their lower extremities. Others contract their erector spinae muscles, sometimes to the point where they extend their lumbar spines.

As described in the preceding section, correction of these motor pattern flaws and facilitation of a symmetrical multifidus activation at the segmental level is accomplished using the principles of motor re-education. The clinician should note that the average patient takes two to three times as long to correctly activate multifidus as they did their transversus abdominis. **It is critical that patients attain each skill level before being progressed to more advanced skills.** Clinicians are strongly encouraged to allow each patient to develop these skills at their own pace. It is a significant management error to assume that greater benefits will be realized by 'skipping' to higher level skills.

Since people are far less aware of their posterior body than their anterior body, the multifidus activation is very difficult. Indeed, it is likely the relatively lower volume of meaningful sensation from the posterior trunk that makes this exercise so difficult. The tactile and verbal feedback provided by the clinician is helpful, and some people respond very well to the tactile input *via* the clinician's finger or thumbs. However, most take significantly longer to learn this activation since they have great difficulty developing any understanding of what it is they are trying to accomplish. Initially, there is very little, if any, of the familiar 'feeling' of a muscle contraction to use as a source of feedback.

The clinician typically notes that the patient learns to activate the multifidus on the unaffected side first with the affected side coming along soon after. As with the initial activation of transversus abdominis, the patient must learn to activate their multifidus at the pathological level, maintain a normal breathing pattern and avoid any contraction of other muscles. The clinical application of various feedback approaches (surface electromyography, pressure biofeedback and ultrasound imaging) designed to assist patients with these exercises is discussed later in this chapter.

Stage Two:
Tonic Hold

Once a patient can independently activate transversus abdominis and multifidus while maintaining a relaxed breathing pattern, they should immediately begin to increase the duration of these activations.

Clinically, it is thought that the maintenance of a tonic activation of these muscles may be necessary to optimally compensate for the underlying increase in neutral zone motion. Therefore the patient is asked to activate their transversus abdominis and multifidus muscles as per the independent activation stage and hold these activations for ten seconds. At this stage, the transversus abdominis and multifidus activations are still performed independent of each other, and of the other trunk muscles. The patient must continue to breathe normally for the duration of the tonic hold. The patient should, with a few days practice, be able to perform ten to fifteen of these activations in succession.

At this point the patient should be instructed to attempt these same activations in other non-weightbearing postures. If the initial activation of transversus abdominis was learned in supine, the patient should begin rehearsing the tonic hold in side-lying (figure 6.22) and eventually, in prone (figure 6.23). The patient should rehearse the isolated tonic hold of their multifidus in the same way. The clinician should advise the patient that as all learning is context specific, these changes in position will result in their transversus abdominis and multifidus activations seeming more difficult. It is anticipated that by learning to activate the transversus abdominis and multifidus in each of supine crook, prone and side-lying, the patient will have developed a higher degree of control of these skills and laid a more complete foundation upon which to access the deep segmental component of their active subsystem in a wider variety of contexts.

Stage Three: Integrated Tonic Hold

Patients invariably demonstrate recruitment patterns in which the superficial multi-segmental muscles are dominant. The objective in the integrated tonic hold stage is to develop the ability to co-activate transversus abdominis and multifidus while minimizing contraction of the superficial, multi-segmental muscles. The patient should eventually be able to perform a series of ten to fifteen second activations in supine, prone and side-lying while breathing normally. This is often most easily learned by the patient if the clinician instructs them to initiate their transversus abdominis activation, maintain it and then add the multifidus activation. Again, supine is a convenient position in which to first facilitate this co-activation using the palpation method described on page 121, whereby the clinician palpates both the ipsilateral transversus abdominis and multifidus (figure 6.24). A higher degree of motor control over this co-activation may be developed later on by rehearsing this pattern in reverse; multifidus is established first, then transversus abdominis is added. Interestingly, some patients automatically activate their transversus abdominis to an appropriate level as they voluntarily activate their multifidus. In such cases it is not necessary to further activate transversus abdominis.

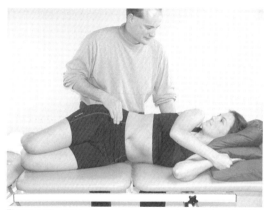

Figure 6.22 Rehearsing the transversus abdominis tonic hold in the side-lying posture.

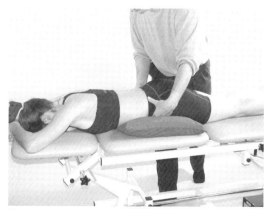

Figure 6.23 Rehearsing the transversus abdominis tonic hold in the prone-lying posture.

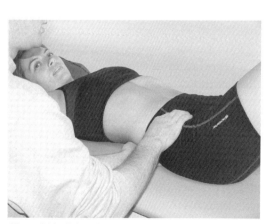

Figure 6.24 Rehearsing the integrated activation of transversus abdominis and multifidus in supine crook-lying.

Stage Four:
Dynamic Activation via Limb Loading

Fourth stage exercises advance both the motor control and mechanical challenges of the third stage skills. The objective is to teach the nervous system to discontinue the compensatory 'bracing-type' contraction of the multi-segmental muscles and to re-establish a more 'selective' pattern. Such a pattern involves the integrated activation of the transversus abdominis and multifidus muscles in combination with the multi-segmental muscles in a context appropriate manner.

The patient is taught to maintain the co-activation of transversus abdominis and multifidus while moving either a lower or an upper extremity through some range of motion. Although the patient remains non-weightbearing, these exercises begin to more closely mimic 'real-life' function as the challenges inherent in maintaining segmental stability and spinal orientation in the presence of upper and lower limb movement are gradually introduced. From a motor control perspective, the neural control subsystem is required to maintain a uniform co-activation of transversus abdominis and multifidus, control the axial and peripheral muscles which will permit the limb to move through range and maintain a normal breathing pattern. From a mechanical perspective, the inertia of the moving limb introduces a low-load segmental stability challenge. The patient must maintain co-activation of transversus abdominis and multifidus as well as a task-appropriate level of contraction of the superficial multi-segmental muscles to maintain the orientation of the lumbar spine against the inertia of the moving limb.

The clinician monitors the posture of the lumbopelvic region, and observes both the patient's breathing pattern and the extent to which their multi-segmental muscles activate relative to transversus abdominis and multifidus (figure 6.25). It is important to note that even with these low load skills, the transversus abdominis and multifidus muscles alone cannot prevent movement of the lumbar spine and pelvis. The mechanical load with such exercises is sufficient to require contraction of the multi-segmental muscles of the trunk to maintain spinal orientation. It must be emphasized that this multi-segmental muscle contraction occurs in addition to, not at the expense of, the co-activation of transversus abdominis and multifidus.

At this stage the clinician's judgment determines whether the degree of multi-segmental muscle activity seems reasonable, given the motor control and mechanical challenges inherent in the exercise. It must be stressed to the patient that the superficial muscles (i.e., the multi-segmental muscles) must not be allowed to dominate the pattern of activation. For example, adequate control of lumbopelvic posture during a relatively low load, lower extremity movement challenge should not require a generalized bracing-type activation of all the trunk muscles. Indeed, this bracing-style activation is the pathologic, compensatory pattern utilized by the neural control subsystem in the presence of segmental pathology; therefore, it is not a pattern clinicians should strive to develop in their patients.

A series of fourth stage exercises are included below. While they are presented in a progressive fashion from easier to more difficult, some variability in their perceived difficulty is to be expected between patients. With each exercise, the patient is instructed to co-activate their transversus abdominis and multifidus and maintain this pattern of activation while moving the upper or lower limb through range. They must continue to breathe normally throughout these exercises.

Supine Posture:
Arm Elevation (figure 6.26)
Bent Knee Fall Out (figure 6.27)
Heel Slide (figure 6.28)

Side-lying Posture:
Hip Abduction (figure 6.29)

Prone Posture:
Knee Flexion (figure 6.30)
Hip Rotation

Supine Posture:
Heel Slide + Arm Elevation

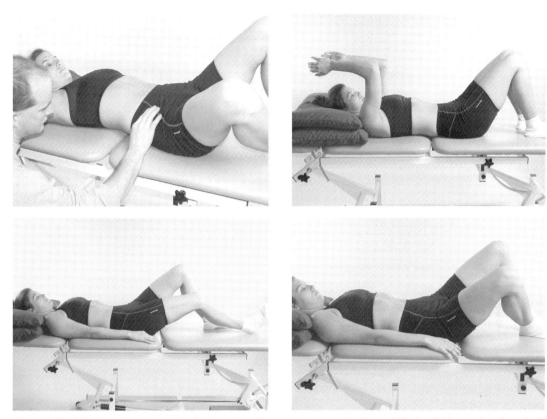

Figures 6.25 - 6.28 Stage Four - Dynamic Limb Loading *Clockwise from upper left:* **Figure 6.25** - the clinician monitors the patient's control of both her lumbopelvic orientation and her lower abdominal wall (transversus abdominis and internal oblique) as she performs a fourth stage exercise. **Figure 6.26** - the patient attempts to maintain a co-contraction of the transversus abdominis and multifidus muscles while moving the arms through elevation. **Figure 6.27** - the patient attempts to maintain a co-contraction of the transversus abdominis and multifidus muscles while allowing a lower extremity to abduct and externally rotate (the 'bent-knee fall-out' exercise). **Figure 6.28** - the patient attempts to maintain a co-contraction of the transversus abdominis and multifidus muscles while allowing a lower extremity to extend along the plinth (the 'heel-slide' exercise).

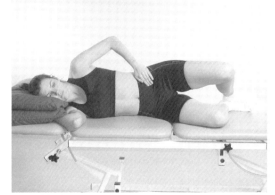

Figure 6.29 The patient attempts to maintain a co-contraction of the transversus abdominis and multifidus muscles while moving the left hip through a small amount of abduction and external rotation.

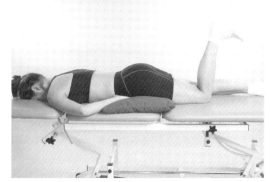

Figure 6.30 The patient attempts to maintain a co-contraction of the transversus abdominis and multifidus muscles while flexing the left knee from the prone posture.

A Therapeutic Dosage of Physiotherapy?

In medicine, the phrase *therapeutic dosage* refers to the minimum amount of drug which must be metabolized by a patient in order to attain a certain therapeutic benefit. In the context of low back pain rehabilitation, no such therapeutic dosage has yet been demonstrated. Using traditional models of spinal rehabilitation, clinicians have come to accept a high degree of uncertainty and unpredictability regarding our patient's responses to traditional therapeutic interventions.

As the authors' approach to therapeutic segmental stabilization exercise has become more homogeneous over the past several years, we have noted that the majority of lumbar patients report a significant and consistent improvement in their symptoms as they are developing good skill with the early or easier fourth stage exercises. This is significant for a variety of reasons. While the authors have utilized other clinical models in the past, we have never before noted such a consistent correlation between the level of exercise skill attained by our patients and the resolution of their symptoms. Significantly, the resolution of symptoms at the fourth stage of the clinical model appears independent of all other factors which might affect rehabilitative outcomes.

There is not a simple timeline correlation since patients begin their rehabilitation at different points in time post onset; some begin the day after their injury, others begin five years after their lumbar spine became symptomatic. Different patients require different amounts of time to learn the exercises and progress through the various stages; while one patient might develop their fourth stage skills in three weeks, another might require seven weeks. Furthermore, this tendency to report a true resolution of symptoms during the fourth stage is independent of diagnosis. While each author approaches the application of this clinical model in a very similar fashion, we do have different clinical and inter-personal styles thus this therapeutic effect seems independent of the clinician applying the treatment. Finally, other clinicians who practice in this fashion report similar outcomes in their patient populations.

Whether or not this represents a true 'therapeutic dosage' remains to be determined through well designed research. Regardless, the authors rarely find it necessary, except with certain patients who will return to competitive sports or a physically demanding occupation, to treat patients beyond the fourth stage of the model. For those lumbar patients who do require stronger muscles and even higher levels of integrated core training, a variety of fifth stage exercises is presented.

Stage Five : Integrative Training

Seated Ball Work (figure 6.31)
Bridging (figure 6.32)
Sport or Work Specific Training

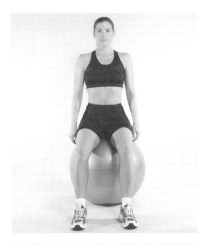

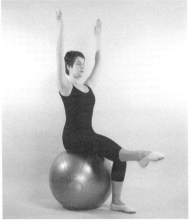

Figure 6.31 Maintaining task-appropriate activation of the trunk muscles with and without perturbations on an unstable surface (from *Jemmett, The Athlete's Ball, 2004* with permission).

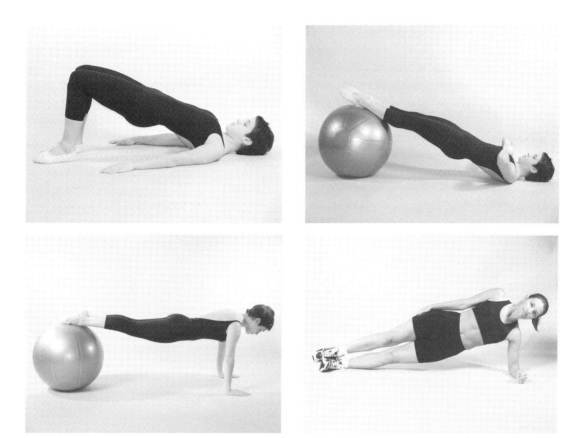

Figures 6.32 A variety of integrative exercises, with and without unstable surfaces. These are complex gross-motor, anti-gravity exercises which should be introduced only after the patient has successfully developed all skills in stages one through four. The increased mechanical and neural control challenges inherent in these exercises are argued to facilitate appropriate integration of the segmental and multi-segmental muscles. This level of mechanical and neural control challenge is most appropriate for patients returning to recreational or occupational activities which place a high demand on the neuromusculoskeletal system. (from *Jemmett, The Athlete's Ball, 2004* with permission).

Biofeedback with Therapeutic Segmental Stabilization Exercises

Pressure Biofeedback Devices

THE PRESSURE BIOFEEDBACK device (PBD) is a modified blood pressure cuff (figure 6.33). It is most appropriately utilized to provide the patient with an understanding of their ability to maintain the orientation of their lumbar spine as they perform fourth stage exercises such as the 'bent knee fall-out' or the 'prone hip rotation'.

The PBD was initially developed as a biofeedback device which could be used to provide both the clinician and the patient with objective evidence of the patient's ability to appropriately

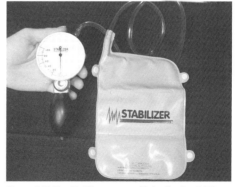

Figure 6.33 The *Stabilizer* pressure biofeedback unit (Chattanooga Group Inc.)

activate their transversus abdominis muscle and to maintain a neutral lumbopelvic posture during fourth stage exercises incorporating movement in the extremities (Richardson et al., 1999).

To monitor transversus abdominis activation, the patient was placed in prone with the PBD under their lower abdomen. With the PBD's air bladder inflated to 70 mm Hg, the patient was asked to draw in their lower abdomen to recruit the transversus abdominis. The patient was asked to draw in sufficiently so as to create an 6 - 10 mm Hg drop in pressure. This drop in pressure was considered evidence of the activation of transversus abdominis (Richardson et al., 1999). However, the 'drawing-in' maneuver is no longer considered an appropriate means of independently activating transversus abdominis as it tends to cause activation of internal oblique; such a large drop in pressure is virtually impossible to achieve using only the transversus abdominis muscle.

Clinically, the monitoring of multifidus activations using the PBD has become common; however, this has proved problematic. Typically, the patient was positioned in supine crook-lying with the PBD, inflated to 40 mm Hg, placed under their lumbopelvic region. The patient was then asked to activate transversus abdominis and multifidus and create an increase of 4 - 6 mm Hg. If the clinician observed a complete absence of lumbopelvic motion, this increase in pressure was taken as evidence of the multifidus muscle activating and 'swelling' outwards, creating greater pressure on the air bladder.

The concern in this regard is twofold. First and foremost, the PBD is unable to selectively monitor the single pathological segment of multifidus which must be monitored and rehabilitated. Assuming that multifidus does expand appreciably as it activates, a patient could very well activate the non-pathological segments of their multifidus, even their longissimus and/or iliocostalis and the PBD would register an increase in pressure. The clinician must use a more segment-specific means of monitoring and facilitating improved activity in the pathological multifidus. Secondly, the increase in pressure may also be developed through a subtle posterior pelvic tilt. Patients who are in-

structed to activate their transversus abdominis and multifidus and create a pressure increase of 4 - 6 mm Hg might instead be moving through a subtle posterior pelvic tilt.

Despite these significant concerns, the PBD does have reasonable clinical application. Once co-activation of transversus abdominis and multifidus has been attained, the PBD may be used to provide the patient with feedback regarding their ability to control the movement of their lumbopelvic region as they perform the various limb-loading skills in the fourth stage. The patient is instructed to activate their transversus abdominis and multifidus and maintain the pressure at a constant level as their limb moves through range. This may be used both in supine crook-lying and prone postures (figures 6.34 and 6.35).

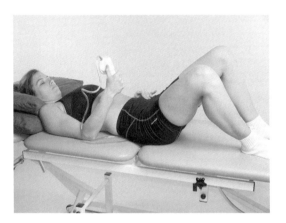

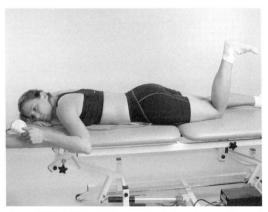

Figure 6.34 & 6.35 The PBD as a tool to help patients monitor their lumbopelvic orientation during various fourth stage exercises. Top - supine 'bent-knee fall-out'. Bottom - prone knee flexion.

Diagnostic or 'Real-Time' Ultrasound Biofeedback

REAL-TIME ULTRASOUND (US) imaging has been utilized to visualize the abdominal wall and the multifidus muscle while patients learn their independent activation exercises (Richardson et al., 1999b). It is felt that the US image provides the patient and the clinician with a powerful form of feedback, facilitating more accurate performance of the independent activation of the deep segmental muscles. Recently, it has been demonstrated that thickness changes in the transversus abdominis, as measured via US imaging, correlated well with EMG activity (McMeeken et al., 2004; Ferreira et al., 2004). This suggests that, in addition to providing biofeedback to assist in the learning and consistent performance of these exercises, US imaging may be utilized as a measure of the function of the deep segmental muscles.

Surface Electromyography

IN BOTH THE CLINICAL and research environments, surface electromyography (SEMG) is a common yet controversial tool. Although a thorough discussion of this form of biofeedback is beyond the scope of this text, a brief review of certain relevant technical and applied factors, along with a discussion of the limitations of SEMG, is necessary. Physical medicine clinicians interested in a more comprehensive review are directed to the text *Clinical Applications in Surface Electromyography: Chronic Musculoskeletal Pain* (Kasman & Wolf, 2004).

SEMG devices monitor the bioelectrical activity occurring within skeletal muscle as an action potential spreads along motor nerves and through a muscle's conductive membranes. This bioelectrical activity also propagates across a variety of layers and types of tissues, and in all directions, through a mechanism known as volume conduction. Any such signal which reaches the surface of the body may be captured and monitored *via* SEMG.

Through electrodes attached to the skin, a SEMG unit collects the minute voltages generated within active skeletal muscle. Two recording electrodes (positive and negative) and a ground electrode constitute a single SEMG channel. Most modern clinical SEMG devices have two or more channels allowing for multiple muscles to be monitored. The diameter and orientation of the electrodes, as well as the center to center distance between electrodes of any single channel, determine the size of the receptive field for that channel. The receptive field of a SEMG channel is a three dimensional construct including both surface area and depth. Generally, smaller electrodes, aligned parallel to the muscle's fiber orientation and spaced closer together will result in a relatively small receptive field. Larger electrodes, aligned at right angles to the fiber orientation and spaced further apart will create a larger receptive field. A single channel of SEMG will indiscriminately collect all bioelectrical signals within its receptive field; its display will reflect the sum total of these signals (figure 6.36).

Typically, SEMG is used to monitor activity in a superficial muscle using electrodes placed directly over the target muscle. The degree to which we can be certain that the signal collected represents the activity of the target muscle is dependent on a number of factors. The size of the receptive field is one such factor, and as discussed above, the clinician does have some influence over this parameter. However, some percentage of the composite signal reaching the channel's receptive field may have originated in a muscle or muscles other than the intended target. In circumstances where nearby muscles (either adjacent or deep to the muscle of interest) might be active simultaneously with the target muscle, volume conduction can result in 'cross-talk'– the contamination of the overall signal with activity from muscles other than the target muscle (Kasman, 1996).

In a recent report it was found that during isometric gross-motor, anti-gravity efforts, data collected using SEMG electrodes placed over the lumbar multifidus was more representative of activity from the ipsilateral longissimus muscle (Stokes et al., 2003). However, upon review of

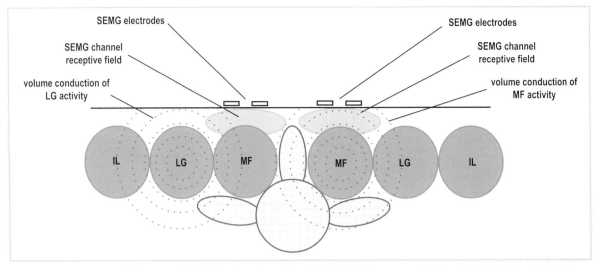

Figure 6.36 The phenomenon of 'volume conduction'. In the above schematic (an inferior 'view' of a transverse section through L4), single channels of SEMG are applied over the right and left multifidus muscles (MF). As shown on the left side, a large percentage of the activity generated by the MF will fall within the receptive field of the SEMG channel overlying the muscle. However, as demonstrated on the opposite side, the longissimus muscle (LG) will also generate a degree of activity likely to fall within the receptive field of the SEMG channel overlying the ipsilateral multifidus. Given that both the MF and the LG (and other muscles as well) may be active ipsilaterally, the resultant signal recorded by a single channel of SEMG will necessarily be a summation of the activity from a number of different muscles.

the data reported by Wolf and colleagues (Wolf et al., 1989), in 16 of the 18 trials presented, both SEMG and intra-muscular electromyography (IEMG) captured similar patterns of activity from the lumbar longissimus muscle during activities including anterior and posterior pelvic tilting, voluntary body sway in standing and shoulder flexion. Although the patterns of activity were very similar, the SEMG tracings were of consistently smaller amplitude than the IEMG tracings. Thus, while volume conduction and the nature of the SEMG receptive field result in concerns regarding cross-talk, SEMG can reflect the activity of its target muscle, although it may tend to underestimate the extent of this activity relative to intra-muscular recordings.

As SEMG is limited in its efficacious application to those muscles found immediately below the skin, it cannot reliably record from muscles such as transversus abdominis, internal oblique or quadratus lumborum. With regard to the multifidus, although it is considered to be a component of the lumbar spine's 'deep' layer, between L3 and S2 it is the most superficial paraspinal muscle found immediately lateral to the spinous processes. However, given the connective

tissues superficial to the multifidus muscle as well as the close proximity of the longissimus muscle, it remains controversial as to whether SEMG can selectively record activity in multifidus. Despite these valid concerns, there remains a reasonable protocol by which SEMG may be utilized clinically to provide patients with enhanced feedback regarding their ability to differentially activate both the transversus abdominis and multifidus muscles.

Independent Activation of Transversus Abdominis using SEMG Biofeedback

Although SEMG cannot selectively record from the transversus abdominis muscle, it can record from muscles such as rectus abdominis and external oblique. If a patient has an unusual amount of difficulty minimizing contraction of their rectus abdominis and/or external oblique while trying to activate the transversus abdominis, the clinician may use SEMG to provide the patient with further information regarding the activation of their superficial abdominal muscles. Clinically, this additional feedback appears to be useful in helping patients learn to minimize unwanted muscle con-

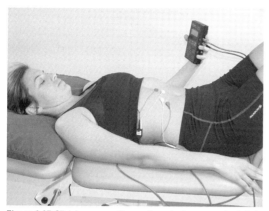

Figure 6.37 Clinicians may utilize surface electromyography to help patients learn to minimize contraction of multi-segmental muscles such as rectus abdominis and external oblique while developing activation of transversus abdominis.

traction. The patient is instructed to activate their transversus abdominis, as described previously, and to minimize any contraction of the rectus abdominis and/or external oblique as per the data on the SEMG display (figure 6.37). Most modern clinical SEMG units monitor two muscles simultaneously and provide both visual and audio feedback. Similar approaches could be developed to assist the patient in developing differential activity of the transversus abdominis relative to other superficial trunk muscles, as indicated.

Independent Activation of Multifidus Using SEMG Biofeedback

As mentioned previously, learning to differentially activate the multifidus muscle is typically quite difficult. While tactile and verbal feedback are helpful, patients initially describe a frustrating lack of 'internal' awareness or feeling of any multifidus muscle contraction. Many patients state they simply "can't feel" the multifidus at all, making it difficult to learn the required skill of initial activation. This may lead to prolonged and potentially less successful rehabilitation. In this situation, provided that certain steps are taken to optimize muscle specificity and minimize cross-talk from nearby muscles, SEMG can be extremely

helpful for patients in the initial activation stage of their multifidus rehabilitation. A patient with a segmental dysfunction at L4-5, symptomatic on the right side, is used to illustrate this technique.

With the patient in prone-lying and using a two-channel SEMG unit, a bilateral set-up is used with one channel over the left L4-5 multifidus and the other over the right (figure 6.38). The electrodes are applied within one centimeter of the midline and the center-to-center distance between the recording electrodes is approximately two centimeters. The gain or sensitivity of the unit should be set so as to ensure an appropriate display of data. In the author's experience, the very subtle contractions developed with correct performance of this exercise requires the sensitivity to be set as high as is available on most SEMG units. At these sensitivity levels, correct performance of the exercise typically results in a display reading of 30 to 50%. It is critical that both the clinician and the patient understand that developing significant activity in the multifidus is NOT the objective of this exercise. Rather, the patient is attempting to differentially activate their multifidus muscle, adjacent to the dysfunctional segment, relative to the other trunk muscles. The degree of activation is of little significance whereas the ability to activate the multifidus while minimizing activity in other trunk muscles is key.

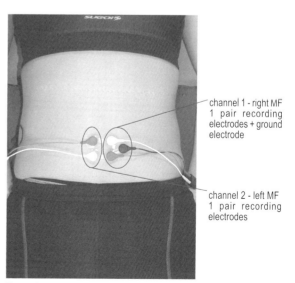

channel 1 - right MF 1 pair recording electrodes + ground electrode

channel 2 - left MF 1 pair recording electrodes

Figure 6.38 Two-channel SEMG set-up over the multifidus muscles at the L4-5 motion segment.

With the electrodes applied, the patient may be repositioned to either supine crook or side-lying, or if preferred, they may remain in prone (use caution with the prone position as few patients are able to tolerate this posture for more than a few minutes). The patient is then taught the first stage independent activation technique for the multifidus, as described previously. The patient and clinician may both observe the SEMG display as the patient attempts to activate their multifidus bilaterally while minimizing contraction in other trunk muscles (figure 6.39). The clinician should also observe the patient's breathing pattern and monitor their trunk *via* palpation for evidence of muscle contraction in adjacent muscles. Lastly, the clinician should compare their palpatory findings regarding the patient's ability to differentially activate the lumbar multifidus (in this case at the right L4-5) with the SEMG data. If there is good correspondence between the SEMG data and palpation, with both indicating activity in the target multifidus muscle, the patient may be allowed to use SEMG as an adjunct source of feedback along with the clinician's verbal and tactile input.

Once the patient appears able to symmetrically activate the bilateral L4-5 multifidus, the two-channel SEMG unit can be used to further develop the patient's skill at activating the multifidus muscle adjacent to the dysfunctional segment independent of other ipsilateral trunk muscles. As our sample patient has a right sided dysfunction with a loss of multifidus volume on the right, we will assume that their ability to differentially activate their right multifidus will be most compromised. Thus, one channel of SEMG will remain at the right L4-5 multifidus while the second channel is set up over the latissimus dorsi and thoracic erector spinae on the right side (figure 6.40). The patient is now instructed to gently activate the multifidus while minimizing contraction of these multi-segmental muscles (MSM). With practice, the patient should be able to demonstrate activation of the multifidus with only negligible contraction of the MSM (figure 6.41). Again, the clinician must monitor the patient's multifidus and MSM *via* both SEMG and palpation, checking for the degree of correspondence between these monitoring tools. Once the patient appears able to activate the right L4-5 multifidus while maintaining a negligible contraction of the MSM, the second channel may be placed over the right longissimus muscle (figure 6.42). The patient is then instructed to activate the multifidus while limiting contraction of the longissimus muscle. If the clinician wishes, they may also palpate whichever of the MSM or longis-

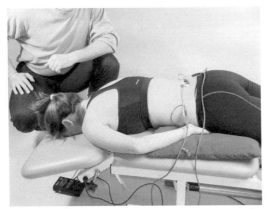

Figure 6.39 The patient observes the SEMG as they learn to differentially activate the multifidus muscle adjacent to their dysfunctional segment. Both patient and clinician can observe the SEMG; the patient palpates transversus abdominis while the clinician is free to observe and/or palpate the patient for signs of co-contraction of the multi-segmental muscles.

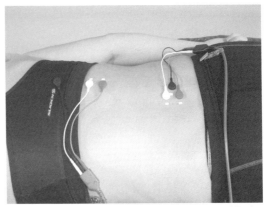

Figure 6.40 SEMG application monitoring the ipsilateral lumbar multifidus muscle and thoracic multi-segmental muscles on the right side. In the above photo, the patient is in prone-lying; however, with the electrodes in place they may rehearse this skill in a variety of postures.

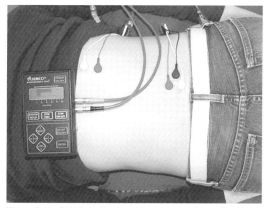

Figure 6.41 SEMG application with one channel over the lumbar multifidus (MF) muscle and the second channel over the ipsilateral multi-segmental muscles (MSM) on the right side. Note the SEMG unit's display - the patient is able to minimize activity in the MSM while activating the MF adjacent to the segmental level of dysfunction.

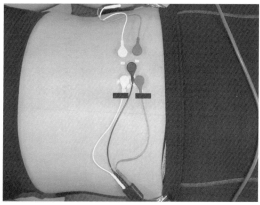

Figure 6.42 SEMG application with one channel over the lumbar multifidus muscle and the second channel over the ipsilateral longissimus on the right side. The bars represent the locations of the L4 and L5 spinous processes.

gravity exercises, bioelectrical signals generated in muscles other than the multifidus will be recorded *via* SEMG electrodes placed over the multifidus. However, as applied using the above protocol, muscle activations are extremely subtle relative to the isometric, whole body efforts studied by Stokes and colleagues (Stokes et al., 2003). As such the amplitudes of the resultant bioelectrical signals are relatively small, and may be screened for. Using observation, palpation and SEMG, the clinician is able to compare the degree of multifidus activity to that of the thoracic MSM, the longissimus and other superficial trunk muscles, minimizing the potential for misinterpretation of the SEMG data.

In our clinical experience, the use of SEMG biofeedback during the initial activation stage of multifidus rehabilitation has shown excellent utility. Patients consistently report the additional feedback to have been extremely helpful, with some describing it as a necessary tool. Given the inherent difficulty in learning to differentially activate the multifidus, patients may experience a degree of 'performance anxiety' in the situation where they are being asked to rehearse the exercise with the clinician observing and/or palpating their trunk muscles for the duration of a treatment session. Once the clinician is satisfied that there is good correspondence between their palpatory appreciation of multifidus activity and the SEMG data, the patient can work independently of the clinician. With skilled facilitation and coaching, this process may require anywhere from two to six treatment sessions to achieve differential activation of the multifidus muscle.

Clinical Coaching Skill as a Prognosis-Modifying Factor

Manual therapy clinicians are often very concerned with skill development in terms of joint assessment and treatment. Many are willing to invest much time, effort and money in acquiring new and more advanced joint mobilization and manipulation techniques and the latest in therapeutic exercise. In the authors' opinion, relatively little attention is paid to our skill at teaching or coaching; papers

simus is not being monitored by the second channel to further ensure a differential activation of the target multifidus muscle.

As discussed previously, there are valid concerns regarding the efficacy of SEMG applications with the lumbar multifidus. Especially important is the potential for activity in other muscles to be mistakenly interpreted as multifidus activity. With muscles such as latissimus dorsi, the gluteals and the erector spinae all having attachments through the connective tissues overlying the lower lumbar multifidus, it is likely that during gross-motor, anti-

and courses on this important clinical topic are few and far between.

In a previous section, the patient's motor skills were described as a significant factor affecting their prognosis. While this is an accurate statement, it is critical that clinicians appreciate that their ability to coach clients through the rehabilitative process in general, and the therapeutic segmental stability exercises in particular, will play a much greater role in influencing the outcome of their treatment. A clinician's ability to facilitate these exercises has far more impact on their patient's prognosis than does the patient's underlying motor skill. Clinicians can expect that as their skills in these methods improve, fewer of their patients will be deemed 'unable' to learn these exercises.

Neurodynamic Treatment Techniques

THE IDEA THAT INJURED osseoligamentous structures can influence pain and lead to a loss of AROM is certainly familiar to clinicians. The same can be said of chemically irritated or mechanically compromised neural tissues. What may be less familiar to clinicians is that impaired mobility of neural tissue, or adverse neurodynamics, can become a significant clinical factor in the setting of a segmental hypomobility and that these neural tissues may be selectively mobilized as a means of improving the patient's physiological ROM.

Once the nervous tissue has been determined to be an active component of the patient's presentation, specific mobilization techniques are utilized to reduce the sensitivity of the nervous tissue to mechanical tension and significantly improve a patient's movement and symptoms. The neurodynamic assessment techniques described in chapter four can also be used as effective treatment techniques in patients whose lumbar dysfunction involves either chemical or mechanical irritation of the neural tissue.

Principles of Mobilization of Neural Tissues in the Lower Quadrant

Mobilization of lower quadrant neural tissues is indicated in two clinical situations. In the first circumstance, the lumbar segmental dysfunction leading to the adverse neurodynamics has been significantly improved *via* articular and therapeutic exercise interventions yet some loss of nervous system mobility persists. In the second, the patient presents with no significant segmental movement dysfunction but rather a chemical irritation of the nervous tissue which perpetuates their adverse neurodynamics.

The clinical guidelines regarding mobilization of the neural tissues are similar to those for mobilization of the passive elements of a motion segment. The amount of mechanical tension applied to the nervous system should correlate with the level of irritability of the nervous system. If, when applying a tensile load to the neural tissues of the lower quadrant, the clinician appreciates only minimal resistance, yet the patient experiences a significant increase in their symptoms, the clinician should assume this to be a highly irritable nervous system that would respond poorly to the application of any additional mechanical force. It is the authors' opinion that, in the case of a patient with a known lumbar dysfunction, it is often best to manage the spinal dysfunction creating the irritation of the nervous tissue and use neurodynamic tests (chapter five) as outcome measures rather than as treatment techniques.

The type of neuromobilization advocated by the authors is argued to apply a tensile force to one end of the nervous system while reducing the tension on the other. This permits nervous tissue movement relative to its interfaces without excessive, and potentially harmful, tensile forces being applied to the nervous tissue. This movement could also enhance circulation to the nervous tissue as well as help remove any associated inflammatory exudates from the site of the neural compromise. The pattern of movement should be such that it specifically biases the component of the nervous system in the lower quadrant which was determined to be irritable in the assessment.

For example, if the slump test, biased to the tibial nerve, demonstrated a neurogenic response during the initial assessment, and the above criteria for neuromobilization were met, then a 'slider' (Butler, 2000) for the tibial nerve may be utilized. The patient will assume a sitting position with their trunk and cervical spine in a flexed position. The patient will then simultaneously dorsiflex and evert their ankle and foot, extend the knee, trunk and cervical spine. In doing so, tension is decreased in the proximal portion of the nervous system and increased in the distal. This is reversed and the patient assumes the start position. The patient is instructed to move as far as they feel comfortable. It is essential that there is no increase in symptoms during this movement. The clinician can expect the patient to experience a physiological response to stretch - a gentle tension in the lower limb for example - but certainly no pain or reports of increased symptoms. This movement is typically repeated ten times and the patient is instructed to perform this movement frequently throughout the day. As mentioned above, the transference of neural tension is hypothesized to generate movement of the nervous tissue without excessively tensioning it. This symptom free movement of the nervous system has frequently demonstrated substantial and immediate improvements in the patient's movement patterns as well as their symptoms.

These concepts can be utilized with any of the neurodynamic tests discussed in this text. The slump version was outlined as this technique allows for the greatest amount of trunk movement and therefore the greatest amount of neural 'sliding' to occur. The SLR can be used as well with the patient making use of extension of the cervical spine to decrease the tension on the nervous system proximally while utilizing knee flexion to decrease the tension distally.

Indwelling Electrical Muscle Stimulation (IEMS)

Indwelling Electrical Muscle Stimulation, as described in this section, has not as yet undergone any form of scientific evaluation. Thus, all comments regarding technique and expected outcomes are based solely on the authors' clinical experience. This intervention is invasive and therefore involves risks similar to those associated with acupuncture. Clinicians must ensure that IEMS falls within their legislated scope of practice prior to utilizing it in clinical practice.

There is considerable evidence, as reviewed in chapter three, that the lumbar multifidus has a significant role to play in the maintenance of spinal stability and the control of neutral zone motion. Furthermore, the lumbar multifidus has been shown, *via* numerous studies, to undergo a loss of volume or cross sectional area adjacent to the pathological segment. Given the current evidence, a reasonable clinical interpretation of this literature is that the multifidus is segmentally dysfunctional in patients with low back pain.

The authors have developed a variation on an existing therapeutic intervention known as indwelling electrical muscle stimulation (IEMS). Using two standard acupuncture needles as electrodes along with an electrical muscle stimulator (EMS) the needle electrodes are inserted directly into the multifidus muscle adjacent and ipsilateral to the dysfunctional lumbar segment. Using a frequency of 3 to 5 Hz, and an intensity sufficient to generate a comfortable degree of contraction, the multifidus muscle is stimulated for 10 to 15 minutes. The objective of this therapeutic intervention is to improve the quality of segmental motion by altering the activation patterns of the lumbar multifidus.

In a majority of our patients, clinical markers such as AROM, combined movement tests, the Slump test and the patient's ratings of pain are markedly improved, either immediately, or within 24 hours of application. We have also observed improvements in the patient's ability to activate the lumbar multifidus in co-activation with the transversus abdominis following application of this intervention.

The authors recognize two potential mechanisms by which these clinical changes might occur. It is possible that electrical stimulation of the segmental multifidus may enhance the recovery of the muscle's function at the dysfunctional segment when provided in conjunction with a rehabilitation program for the segmental stabilizing muscles. Alternatively, electrical stimulation may alter the neurophysiological characteristics of the multifidus muscle, and perhaps the segment itself, leading to more normal muscle tone and more functional segmental mechanics.

Suitable Patients

Patients who present with unilateral low back pain, evidence of an isolated segmental dysfunction, a unilateral decrease in multifidus cross sectional area, and an increase in segmental compliance should respond well to this technique. Patients with bilateral signs and symptoms and/or decreases in segmental movement and compliance do not tend to respond as favourably. Importantly, the patient should not have any appreciable apprehension about the use of needles or any other aspect of the technique.

Technique

The patient is positioned comfortably in side-lying so that their symptomatic side is 'up' and the patient's lumbar spine is in a neutral position. Pillows, towel rolls, etc., are used as needed to ensure patient comfort. Alternatively, the patient may be positioned in prone if the clinician is confident that this posture will be well tolerated. The technique, its anticipated therapeutic effect, and all cautions and contraindications are made known to the patient such that they may give their informed consent to the intervention.

With the pathological segment identified *via* a thorough examination, two acupuncture needles (.22 X 40 mm) are inserted one to two centimeters lateral to the midline adjacent and ipsilateral to the involved segment. The needles are inserted

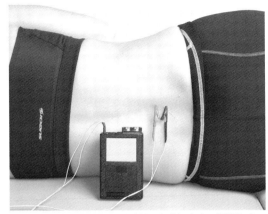

Figure 6.43 Indwelling Electrical Muscle Stimulation (IEMS). Acupuncture needles function as electrodes and are inserted into the multifidus muscle adjacent to the dysfunctional segment. Above, the right L4-5 multifidus is treated. See text for details regarding technique, cautions and contraindications.

such that they 'bracket' the dysfunctional segment (along a cranial to caudal orientation) and are no greater than two centimeters apart. The needle electrodes are inserted such that a minimum of five millimeters of needle remains outside the body; the depth of insertion is tailored to suit the relative size of the patient and the anticipated depth of their multifidus muscle. 'Alligator clip' extensions are used to attach the leads of a standard* EMS unit to the exposed length of each needle electrode (figure 6.43).

The stimulation parameters are set as follows:

• frequency 3 - 5 Hz
• output - 100% per channel
• ramp - 1 second
• on time - 10 seconds
• off time - 10 seconds

With the needle electrodes in place, the patient should be asked if they remain comfortable; if so, the clinician turns the EMS unit on and gradually increases the unit's output (intensity) until a muscle twitch is observed or the patient reports that they have reached their tolerance level. The treatment may last from ten to fifteen minutes. When the treatment is completed, the EMS unit is turned off and the needle electrodes removed

---

*Clinicians are strongly advised to conduct a self-test of any EMS device prior to providing this intervention to their patients. Ensure the unit works correctly and that the indwelling stimulation can be made comfortable prior to application.

from the patient and disposed of in the appropriate fashion.

Cautions and Contraindications

The expected complications associated with IEMS include all known or anticipated risks and complications associated with acupuncture and electro-acupuncture. As such, the most common complications are small bleeds, haematomas and pain during insertion or removal of the needle electrode. Orthostatic dysregulation (fainting) during lumbar IEMS is expected to occur rarely, if at all, as patients will be lying down during treatment. Infection transmission during IEMS is a possible complication; however, the use of pre-sterilized, single-use needles along with appropriate skin preparation greatly diminishes any risk of infection. Concerns regarding potential CNS-related risks secondary to the application of electrical currents across the spinal column have been raised. These concerns pertain to a single channel of EMS applied across the midline with the positive and negative electrodes inserted into muscles on opposite sides of the spine. This is a non-issue with lumbar IEMS as the needle electrodes of a given IEMS channel remain ipsilateral to the spine.

The following is a comprehensive although non-exhaustive list of cautions and contraindications to lumbar IEMS:

Absolute Contraindications

- pacemakers
- imbedded neural stimulators
- pregnancy
- seizure disorders
- patients who express any apprehension regarding any aspect of the intervention
- any patient whom the clinician suspects may have an as yet undiagnosed fracture

Relative Contraindications

- wound-healing disorders
- immunosuppressive disorders
- coagulation defects including blood thinning medications
- valvular heart disease

Cautions

- any patient whom the clinician suspects may have an acute disc herniation
- IEMS may over-sedate older patients causing risk of falling asleep after treatment; the clinician may wish to ensure that elderly patients have made arrangements to be driven home following their appointment

Expected Outcome

Immediately following IEMS treatment, the patient should be re-examined, testing their restricted combined movement, and, if positive on initial examination, their neurodynamics. Typically, significant improvements in range of motion and pain will be observed, either immediately or within twenty-four hours of treatment.

This intervention should not be utilized more than three times with the same patient. IEMS is expected to affect only a transient change in the dysfunctional multifidus muscle. It is not anticipated to be capable of restoring normal function of the neuromuscular system. Thus, therapeutic exercises must be performed in order to rehabilitate the active subsystem and achieve a more complete correction of the patient's problem. As with manipulation, clinicians should be aware of the limitations of these techniques, and the need for a comprehensive management plan.

Clinical Patterns of Segmental Dysfunction: Findings, Clinical Impression, Prognosis & Management

Chapter four presented an overview of four primary categories or sub-groups of segmental dysfunction. These four sub-groups may be expanded to account for the wide variety of patient presentations encountered in clinical practice. The following twelve patterns of segmental dysfunction present the key findings, prognosis and suggested management for each clinical pattern. The assessment techniques utilized to arrive at the clinical impressions listed below are discussed throughout chapter five.

Segmental Dysfunction Pattern 1

Key Findings:
- increased uni-planar segmental compliance isolated to a single lumbar segment
- decreased volume of the multifidus muscle adjacent to the dysfunctional segment
- normal segmental compliance elsewhere in the lumbar spine, pelvis or hips
- normal or abnormal neurodynamics
- normal neurological screening examination

Impression:
A single level, uni-directional clinical instability due to pathology (traumatic or non-traumatic) affecting the passive subsystem. The neural control and active subsystems will be impaired secondary to pain and a loss of normal proprioceptive outflow from the pathologic passive subsystem. The degree of this neural control and active subsystem dysfunction is hypothesized to be proportionate to the extent of the laxity in the passive subsystem.

Prognosis:
Good to excellent.

Treatment:
- education regarding diagnosis and prognosis
- therapeutic exercise to improve the function of the segmental stabilizing muscles
- indwelling electrical muscle stimulation at the dysfunctional multifidus muscle
- neurodynamic techniques as indicated

Segmental Dysfunction Pattern 2

Key Findings:
- increased uni-planar segmental compliance isolated to a single lumbar segment
- decreased volume of the multifidus muscle adjacent to the dysfunctional segment
- decreased segmental compliance elsewhere in lumbar spine, pelvis or hips
- normal or abnormal neurodynamics
- normal neurological screening examination

Impression:
A single level clinical instability due to pathology (traumatic or non-traumatic) affecting the passive subsystem in the presence of an excessively stiff segment. The clinically unstable segment is most likely the source of the patient's symptoms. The stiff segment may be non-causal for the clinical instability, while serving to perpetuate it.

Prognosis:
Good to excellent depending the severity of the clinical instability and the degree of stiffness at the adjacent segment.

Treatment:
- education regarding diagnosis and prognosis
- therapeutic exercise to improve the function of the segmental stabilizing muscles
- mobilization or manipulation of the stiff segment if it perpetuates the clinical instability
- indwelling electrical muscle stimulation at the dysfunctional multifidus muscle
- neurodynamic techniques as indicated

Segmental Dysfunction Pattern 3

Key Findings:
- increased uni-planar segmental compliance isolated to a single lumbar segment
- decreased volume of the multifidus muscle adjacent to the dysfunctional segment
- normal segmental compliance elsewhere in the lumbar spine, pelvis and hips
- abnormal neurodynamics
- positive signs on two or more components of the neurological screening examination

Impression:
A single level clinical instability due to pathology (traumatic or non-traumatic) affecting the passive subsystem with nerve root compromise.

Prognosis:
Variable, depending on the severity of the clinical instability and the degree of nerve root compromise.

Treatment:
- education regarding diagnosis, prognosis and alteration of the patients daily activities to avoid further compression or compromise of the nerve root
- therapeutic exercise to improve the function of the segmental stabilizing muscles
- indwelling electrical muscle stimulation at the dysfunctional multifidus muscle
- neurodynamic techniques as indicated

Segmental Dysfunction Pattern 4

Key Findings:
- increased uni-planar segmental compliance isolated to a single lumbar segment
- decreased volume of the multifidus muscle adjacent to the dysfunctional segment
- decreased segmental compliance elsewhere in the lumbar spine, pelvis or hips
- abnormal neurodynamics
- positive signs on two or more components of the neurological screening examination

Impression:
A single level clinical instability due to pathology (traumatic or non-traumatic) affecting the passive subsystem in the presence of an excessively stiff adjacent segment with nerve root compromise (a combination of patterns 2 and 3).

Prognosis:
Variable, depending on the severity of the clinical instability, the degree of stiffness at the adjacent segment and the extent of the nerve root compromise.

Treatment:
- education regarding diagnosis, prognosis and alteration of the patients daily activities to avoid further compression or compromise of the nerve root
- therapeutic exercise to improve the function of the segmental stabilizing muscles
- mobilization or manipulation of the stiff segment if it appears to maintain the clinical instability
- indwelling electrical muscle stimulation at the dysfunctional multifidus muscle
- neurodynamic techniques as indicated

Segmental Dysfunction Pattern 5

Key Findings:
• increased multi-planar segmental compliance isolated to a single lumbar segment
• decreased volume of the multifidus muscle adjacent to the dysfunctional segment
• normal segmental compliance elsewhere in the lumbar spine, pelvis and hips
• normal or abnormal neurodynamics
• normal neurological screening examination

Impression:
A single level, multi-directional clinical instability due to pathology (traumatic or non-traumatic) involving the passive subsystem.

Prognosis:
Poor to moderate depending primarily on the patient's ability to gain a high degree of control of their segmental stabilizing muscles at the dysfunctional segment (the neural control and active subsystems will be markedly impaired secondary to pain and a loss of normal proprioceptive outflow from the pathologic passive subsystem).

Treatment:
• education regarding diagnosis and prognosis
• therapeutic exercise to improve the function of the segmental stabilizing muscles
• indwelling electrical muscle stimulation at the dysfunctional multifidus muscle
• neurodynamic techniques as indicated

Segmental Dysfunction Pattern 6

Key Findings:
• increased multi-planar segmental compliance isolated to a single lumbar segment
• decreased volume of the multifidus muscle adjacent to the dysfunctional segment
• decreased segmental compliance elsewhere in the lumbar spine, pelvis or hip
• normal or abnormal neurodynamics
• normal neurological screening examination

Impression:
A single level, multi-directional clinical instability due to pathology (traumatic or non-traumatic) affecting the passive subsystem in the presence of an excessively stiff adjacent segment.

Prognosis:
Poor to moderate pending the patient's ability to develop excellent control of their segmental stabilizing muscles at the dysfunctional segment. Also variable is the extent to which the stiff segment is 'driving' the clinical instability and the degree to which the stiff segment will respond to treatment.

Treatment:
• education regarding the severity of the dysfunction and the prognosis is essential in such patients as any significant change in their condition will take considerable time and effort; realistic goals must be established at the time of the initial evaluation
• therapeutic exercise to improve the function of the segmental stabilizing muscles
• indwelling electrical muscle stimulation at the dysfunctional multifidus muscle
• manipulate or mobilize the adjacent stiff segment if it appears to perpetuate the clinical instability
• neurodynamic techniques as indicated

Segmental Dysfunction Pattern 7

Key Findings:
- increased multi-planar segmental compliance isolated to a single lumbar segment
- decreased volume of the multifidus muscle adjacent to the dysfunctional segment
- normal segmental compliance elsewhere in the lumbar spine, pelvis and hips
- abnormal neurodynamics
- positive signs on two or more components of the neurological screening examination

Impression:
Likely a significant multi-directional clinical instability with nerve root compromise.

Prognosis:
Poor, depending on the degree of nerve root compromise and the patient's ability to gain excellent control of their segmental stabilizing muscles. Such patients are likely to require surgical consultation.

Treatment:
- education regarding the severity of the dysfunction and the prognosis is essential in such patients as any significant change in their condition will take considerable time and effort; realistic goals must be established at the time of the initial evaluation; instruction regarding the modification of their daily activities so as to avoid further compromise of the nerve root is also required
- therapeutic exercise to improve the function of the segmental stabilizing muscles
- indwelling electrical muscle stimulation is used with caution given the possibility that any abrupt change in local muscle tone may exacerbate the patient's status
- neurodynamic techniques will likely be *contraindicated* in such cases since any degree of mechanical load applied to the neural tissues is likely to exacerbate the patient's symptoms

Segmental Dysfunction Pattern 8

Key Findings:
- increased multi-planar segmental compliance isolated to a single lumbar segment
- decreased volume of the multifidus muscle adjacent to the dysfunctional segment
- decreased segmental compliance elsewhere in the lumbar spine, pelvis and hips
- abnormal neurodynamics
- positive signs on two or more components of the neurological screening examination

Impression:
A single level, multi-directional clinical instability due to pathology (traumatic or non-traumatic) affecting the passive subsystem in the presence of an excessively stiff adjacent segment with nerve root compromise. A significant loss of passive subsystem function is suggested by this presentation.

Prognosis:
Very poor. Such patients require further medical investigation and a surgical consult. Physiotherapeutic intervention of any form will frequently be of little value in patients with this degree of dysfunction.

Treatment:
- education regarding the severity of the dysfunction and the prognosis is essential; instruction regarding the modification of daily activities so as to avoid further compromise of the nerve root
- therapeutic segmental stabilization exercise
- indwelling electrical muscle stimulation is used with caution - any abrupt change in local muscle tone may exacerbate the patient's status
- neurodynamic techniques will likely be *contraindicated* as any degree of mechanical load applied to the neural tissues is likely to exacerbate the patient's symptoms
- mobilize the adjacent stiff segment if it perpetuates the clinical instability and only if the patient can tolerate this intervention without exacerbation of their symptoms

Segmental Dysfunction Pattern 9

Key Findings:
- **decreased uni-planar segmental compliance isolated to a single segment**
- **decreased volume of the multifidus muscle adjacent to the dysfunctional segment**
- normal segmental compliance elsewhere in the lumbar spine, pelvis or hips
- normal or abnormal neurodynamics
- normal neurological screening examination

Impression:
The above findings may develop secondary to one of two distinct mechanisms:

1. Older adult with radiographic evidence of moderate to advanced osteoarthritis and degenerative disc disease.
   - despite decreased segmental compliance at the symptomatic segment, segmental stabilizing muscle function will still be impaired secondary to a loss of normal proprioceptive outflow from the pathologic segment

2. Younger patient with underlying segmental dysfunction overlaid with excessive multi-segmental muscle activity resulting in a 'compressed' joint.
   - this segmental dysfunction involves an apparent decrease in compliance (a very stiff segment); however, on examination it is appreciated that the segment actually is excessively compliant, the high level of stiffness is secondary to excessive multi-segmental muscle activity (guarding)

Prognosis:
1. moderate to good depending on the extent of degenerative changes and other co-existent health conditions (e.g., diabetes mellitus, peripheral vascular disease)

2. good to excellent depending on the extent of the dysfunction and the patient's skill with segmental stabilizing exercises

Treatment:
- education regarding condition, prognosis, and general activity
- manipulation or mobilization of the stiff segment will often be of value in patients with such findings; encourage patient to perform some form of self-mobilization at home
- therapeutic exercise to improve the function of the segmental stabilizing muscles
- indwelling electrical muscle stimulation at the dysfunctional multifidus muscle
- neurodynamic techniques as indicated

Segmental Dysfunction Pattern 10

Key Findings:
- decreased uni-planar segmental compliance at two or more lumbar segments
- decreased volume of the multifidus muscle adjacent to the dysfunctional segments
- decreased segmental compliance elsewhere in the lumbar spine, pelvis or hips
- normal or abnormal neurodynamics
- normal neurological screening examination

Impression:
Multi-level moderate to advanced osteoarthritis and/or degenerative disc disease. Despite decreased segmental compliance at the symptomatic segment, segmental stabilizing muscle function will still be impaired because of the loss of normal proprioceptive outflow from the pathologic segment.

Prognosis:
Moderate depending on the severity of the degenerative changes and other co-existent health conditions (e.g., diabetes mellitus, peripheral vascular disease).

Treatment:
- education regarding condition, prognosis, and general activity
- manipulation or mobilization of the stiff segments will often be of value in patients with such findings; encourage patient to perform some form of self-mobilization at home
- therapeutic exercise to improve the function of the segmental stabilizing muscles
- indwelling electrical muscle stimulation at the dysfunctional multifidus muscle
- neurodynamic techniques as indicated

Segmental Dysfunction Pattern 11

Key Findings:
- decreased uni-planar segmental compliance isolated to a single segment
- decreased volume of the multifidus muscle adjacent to the dysfunctional segment
- normal segmental compliance elsewhere in the lumbar spine, pelvis and hips
- abnormal neurodynamics
- positive findings on neurological screening examination

Impression:
These findings are indicative of spinal stenosis.

Prognosis:
Poor to good depending on the severity and location of the stenotic changes and the presence of other co-existent health conditions (e.g., osteoarthritis, diabetes mellitus, peripheral vascular disease). Surgery may be indicated in more severe presentations.

Treatment:
In the case of a lateral recess stenosis, mobilization may be helpful in lessening the mechanical compression of the nerve root. By increasing the compliance associated with flexion at the segment, intervertebral foramen diameter may be increased thereby decreasing the mechanical compression of the nerve root. Techniques to improve flexion and side bending on the stenotic side are often utilized with variable success in terms of symptom modification. In the case of a central stenosis the potential for improvement in the patient's condition is markedly reduced.
- improved function of the segmental stabilizing muscles may restore some measure of segmental motion control
- indwelling electrical muscle stimulation at the dysfunctional multifidus muscle is an option; however, in practice this seems to be of limited value in such presentations
- neurodynamic techniques may be utilized if a reasonable degree of symptom relief has been attained *via* mobilization

Segmental Dysfunction Pattern 12

Key Findings:
- decreased segmental compliance isolated to a single segment
- decreased segmental compliance elsewhere in the lumbar spine, pelvis and hips
- abnormal neurodynamics
- positive signs on two or more components of the neurological screening examination

Impression:
These findings are indicative of marked degenerative changes in the vertebral column including significant nerve root compromise. Central and lateral recess stenosis are likely components of this presentation.

Prognosis:
Poor to moderate depending on the extent and location of the stenotic changes and the presence of other co-existent health conditions (e.g., osteoarthritis, diabetes mellitus, peripheral vascular disease). Surgery may be indicated in more severe presentations.

Treatment:
- education regarding the severity of the dysfunction and the prognosis is essential in such patients; instruction regarding the modification of their daily activities so as to avoid further compromise of the nerve root is also required
- gentle mobilization techniques can be utilized at the stiff segments with the emphasis placed on self mobilization
- improved function of the segmental stabilizing muscles may restore some measure of segmental motion control
- indwelling electrical muscle stimulation is used with caution given the possibility that any abrupt change in local muscle tone may exacerbate the patient's status
- neurodynamic mobilization will likely be *contraindicated* as any mechanical load applied to the neural tissues is likely to result in an exacerbation of the patient's symptoms

Summary

This chapter has described a wide range of physiotherapeutic interventions which may be utilized to manage patients with symptoms suggestive of lumbar segmental dysfunction. As in all circumstances, the interventions chosen to manage any single patient must be in keeping with the clinician's legislated scope of practice and individual skill set and should be selected upon a thorough appreciation for the specific features of the patient's segmental dysfunction. Many of the techniques presented require the clinician to undertake further education to ensure safe and efficacious application. The twelve patterns of lumbar segmental dysfunction described at the end of the chapter are presented to assist clinicians in developing an understanding of the relationships between key findings, prognosis and management. While these twelve patterns will account for a significant portion of the patients encountered in clinical practice, further refinements and additions to this set should be anticipated.

The final chapter takes our discussion of prospective clinical reasoning, the segmental dysfunction model and clinical patterns from the theoretical to the practical *via* a thorough examination of ten case studies representing actual patients as treated by the authors.

clinical case studies

The intent of this chapter is to integrate the scientific and clinical information presented in this text. We hope to demonstrate, in a highly practical manner, an evidence-based, best-practice rationale for the management of patients with lumbar dysfunction. We have structured these case studies using a strong clinical reasoning model which will help the reader appreciate the efficacy in the assessment and treatment approaches discussed in previous chapters.

These case studies are taken from each author's clinical practice. In all cases, each patient gave their informed consent to treatment. Each patient's goal of treatment was a reduction in pain and an ability to return to their normal activities as related to daily living, occupation and sport or fitness pursuits.

Case Study 1 (Jemmett)

Subjective Examination:

34 year old single female without children. She worked as an administrator and was a distance runner training for the half-marathon. She reported a long history of episodic lateral right knee pain and distal lateral thigh pain which co-existed in time. Typically these symptoms were aggravated by running; she stated that the pain had been developing earlier in her runs (at about the 8 km mark). She noted also that her pain could be elicited with prolonged walking on hard surfaces. On direct questioning she reported some night time pain, but only when her symptoms were especially bad. Previous history included a menisectomy on the left (the non-symptomatic knee); she denied any history of low back pain.

Objective Examination:

Active movements of the lumbar spine demonstrated greater than normal range into all planes. No symptoms were elicited with lumbar AROM testing. The H & I test demonstrated an asymmetry into the left extension quadrant - she had far greater extension if she moved into extension before side bending. Her extension was very limited if she moved into side bending first. Still no symptoms were elicited. The Slump test elicited a clinical response. PIVMs and SCTs were unremarkable; there was no evidence of hypomobility and no symptoms were reproduced. There was a slight increase in segmental compliance or 'give' with a sidelying anterior-posterior segmental integrity test (APSIT) at L3-4. The patient was able to activate her transversus abdominis appropriately with minimal guidance.

The Ober test was symmetrical bilaterally. On palpation, a marked contraction of the right TFL was noted as the patient attempted to gently abduct the right hip in a left side-lying posture. The right gluteus medius demonstrated a significantly lower degree of activity. There was no such dominance of the TFL when the non-involved side was tested. Likewise there was increased tone of the right TFL as the patient attempted to activate her transversus abdominis via the pelvic floor. The distal ITB was tender on palpation. On palpation, segmental assessment of the lumbar multifidus revealed atrophy at the right L3-4 level.

Working Diagnosis:

This patient had evidence of both a true mechanical lesion at the lateral knee related to abnormal tensioning of the ITB as well as some amount of neurodynamic dysfunction. Both were due to a mild segmental dysfunction or clinical instability at L3-4. The increased tone and inappropriate patterning of the right TFL was interpreted as an attempt by the neural control subsystem to improve lumbopelvic stability, likely along with other muscles which were not, or could not be, assessed *via* palpation. The increased tone in the right TFL likely led to the increased tensioning of her right iliotibial band. The asymmetrical H & I test, the increased compliance noted on the APSIT and the segmental multifidus atrophy directly implicated the lumbar spine in the patient's presentation.

Prognosis:

Good to excellent.

Management and Outcome:

The patient was educated as to the diagnosis and the etiology of her problem. Significant initial treatment time was spent covering all aspects of the origin of her problem as she needed to appreciate the cause of her knee pain if she was to be compliant with an exercise program directed at the lumbar spine. She was told she could continue running but to limit her runs to a distance just less than that at which she typically became symptomatic. When the patient inquired about ITB stretches she was further educated about the cause of her knee pain emphasizing the fact that, while the ITB felt 'tight', it was not truly shortened; the increased tension in the ITB was due to the neural control sub-system's increased activation of the TFL, secondary to the clinical instability at L3-4.

Physiotherapy sessions were dedicated to teaching the patient to improve the function of her SSM system (chapter six, page 116). Following three weeks of intervention at a frequency of two sessions per week, the patient had good activation of both transversus abdominis and multifidus and could effectively perform initial fourth stage exercises. The SSM activation occurred without increased tension in the right TFL as did side-lying hip abduction. At that point, she had noted a decrease in her symptoms and was able to run over 12 km without pain. She was asked to continue her exercises independently and to progress her running as tolerated and at no more than 10% per week. The patient returned for follow-up four weeks later and remained symptom-free at distances of 16 to 18 km; her exercises were well performed. The patient was discharged at this time.

Case Study 2 (Jemmett)

Subjective Examination:

37 year old female, married with two children, aged six and nine. She was a homemaker who attended fitness classes three times per week and performed a muscle endurance training program two to three times per week. She had never been a runner nor a cyclist. She reported a two year history of episodic left inferolateral knee pain, diagnosed most recently as ITB friction syndrome. She stated that her pain was often inconsistent in its presentation and that she was just as likely to be aggravated by a fitness class as she was by sitting for more than twenty minutes. On direct questioning she stated that her pain with sitting could develop even if she had been non-symptomatic just prior to sitting. She also experienced episodes of night time pain which disturbed her sleep.

The patient described a history of chronic low back pain with referral to the posterior left thigh, previously diagnosed as sciatica. She had no previous treatment for either the knee pain nor the 'sciatica' which she had always considered as being two distinct problems.

Objective Examination:

Observation of standing posture revealed an increased lumbar lordosis and tissue creases across the lumbar region at the level of the iliac crests. Lumbar AROM was full and symptom-free; however, it appeared that an inordinate amount of the lumbar movement occurred at approximately the L4-5 level. With movement into extension the patient seemed to 'hinge' at L4-5. Single limb standing was normal on the right; however, on the left the patient internally rotated at the left hip and dropped into a slight Trendelenburg posture. In sitting, left side bending was uncomfortable but full.

The neurological screening examination was normal. The Slump test elicited a neurogenic response on the left side and reproduced her typical lateral left knee pain. This inferolateral knee pain was elicited and abolished with cervical flexion and extension, respectively. On the right, the Slump test elicited posterior thigh tension which was similarly modified with cervical movement. In supine, a modified SLR test (hip adduction with ankle dorsiflexion) elicited the patients primary symptoms.

PIVMs demonstrated relatively increased range into extension at the L4-5 motion segment and SCTs (a cranially directed PA at L5) revealed an increase in connective tissue compliance. The sidelying APSIT demonstrated a marked increase in segmental compliance or 'give' at L4-5. Atrophy of the left multifidus at L4-5 was readily apparent. There was no tenderness along the mid or distal iliotibial band. The patient was able to develop a reasonable transversus abdominis activation *via* the pelvic floor with only a few minutes of coaching.

Working Diagnosis:

L4-5 clinical instability with compromise of the L5 nerve root leading to adverse neurodynamics involving the sciatic and peroneal nerves.

Prognosis:

The patient was thought to have a guardedly optimistic prognosis. While she had only a single-level, uni-directional clinical instability, there was a good degree of increased compliance at the segment. Further, she appeared quite skeptical of the diagnosis in that she had been told by a surgeon that her knee pain was due to ITB syndrome. The fact that she was able to quickly develop reasonable control of her transversus abdominis was positive from a prognostic perspective.

Management and Outcome:

The greatest challenge with this patient was gaining her confidence regarding the diagnosis of clinical instability in the lumbar spine as the cause of her symptoms. She had a difficult time appreciating the fact that a low back problem could cause her lateral knee pain. This necessitated a significant investment of time on education and in demonstrating to the patient the ability of the slump test to reproduce her symptoms.

Treatment consisted entirely of education (regarding fitness classes and sitting duration) and therapeutic exercises to improve the function of her segmental stabilizing system. Shortly after the patient had developed good control of multifidus in both prone and supine she no longer experienced night time nor sitting-related pain. At five weeks she had developed good skill with the fourth stage exercises (the limb-loading tasks) and her exercise program was progressed to include seated stability ball activities. At six weeks the patient's symptoms were controlled during all her normal activities. She was discharged and instructed to maintain her therapeutic exercises at least three times per week for the next several months.

Addendum to Case Studies 1 and 2:

These two case studies (along with David's case study 10) demonstrate the potential for the lumbar spine to be the origin of various peripheral symptoms, previously considered to be independent pathologies of the hip, knee or foot. Examples include piriformis syndrome, greater trochanteric bursitis, ITB friction syndrome, infrapatellar fat pad irritation and plantar fasciitis. While actual pathology may well exist in such local tissues in some situations, there will be a population of patients in whom the causal pathology exists in the lumbar spine and manifests by a variety of mechanisms as peripheral symptoms.

Case Study 3 (Jemmett)

Subjective Examination:

42 year old male, married with one teenage son. He was employed as an automobile mechanic and normally performed a weight training program three to four times per week. He reported a two month history of acute onset low back and anterior left thigh pain which came on suddenly while he was washing dishes. He stated he was unable to tolerate anything other than horizontal positions for the first two weeks of this episode. He described

the location of his pain as being in the lower left back and 'sweeping across' the front of his thigh, continuing to the medial aspect of his left knee. He stated that his leg pain was consistently worse than his back pain. He complained also of a complete numbness of the anterior left thigh. While he had experienced difficulty sleeping secondary to his symptoms for most of the previous two months, in the past week his ability to sleep had been improving. He had not been at work since the onset of his symptoms. He had difficulty descending stairs as he 'didn't trust his left knee' for fear it would give out.

Previous history included several less lengthy episodes of sudden onset low back and leg pain; the leg pain had consistently been worse than the back pain. This patient had Crohn's disease but was otherwise healthy.

Objective Examination:

This gentleman was a large man standing 1.87 m (6'2") and weighing approximately 104 kg (230 lbs). His gait was abnormal in that his left stance time was reduced. Tissue creases were evident at the L4-5 level bilaterally. He did not display any significant protective behaviors as he moved from sitting to standing nor as he moved from sitting to supine on the examination plinth.

Standing lumbar AROM was full and painfree. It appeared that the majority of his lumbar extension occurred at the L4-5 level, consistent with the pattern of tissue creasing. Combined movements were full and comfortable with the exception of left side bending and extension which elicited a sharp 'pinching' sensation near the left posterior superior iliac spine. On H & I testing the patient's movements into the right extension quadrant were symmetrical and not especially symptomatic. Into the left extension quadrant the patient had far less left sidebending if extension was performed first. With extension then left sidebending his previously mentioned 'pinching' sensation was elicited. Single limb standing was quite impaired on the left; the patient appeared to have great difficulty balancing on the left lower extremity.

The patient's L2-3 myotome test demonstrated marked neurogenic weakness. The L3 reflex on the left was less brisk than on the right. Sensation (light touch and pinprick) were altered but not absent over most of the distal anterior left thigh and medial left knee. The supine SLR test elicited a neurogenic response on the left.

SCTs (a cranially directed PA at the L5 spinous process) revealed a significant degree of compliance and reproduced the patient's left PSIS pain. The sidelying APSIT demonstrated increased compliance or give at the L2-3 motion segment relative to L3-4 and markedly increased give at L4-5 relative to L3-4. Palpation of the lumbar paraspinals demonstrated a significant loss of volume throughout most of the multifidus muscle on the left side. The patient was unable to gain independent activation of transversus abdominis on initial assessment.

Working Diagnosis:

A multi-level, unidirectional clinical instability involving the L2-3 and L4-5 motion segments. Significant nerve root compromise, likely secondary to L2-3 intervertebral disc herniation, was also noted.

Prognosis:

Poor to moderate. The patient had had several similar but less dramatic episodes in previous years. Given the current literature it is reasonable to expect that this patient had sustained dysfunction in each of the passive, active and neural control subsystems for several years. The current episode led to significant neurological findings indicative of nerve root compromise and he had two vertebral levels which tested positive for clinical instability. Furthermore, his inability to develop a reasonable transversus abdominis activation on assessment may have been indicative of less than optimal motor control generally.

Management and Outcome:

The patient was educated at length regarding his problem including a comprehensive discussion of the relevant anatomy, motor control and pathology-related issues. A therapeutic segmental stabilization program was initiated as per the discussion in chapter five.

This patient's treatment consisted of 13 sessions over a three month period. Within two treatment sessions, the patient learned to activate his transversus abdominis quite well in supine, side lying and in prone. He was comfortable in the prone position thus initial efforts to voluntarily activate the multifidus were commenced in this posture. By the fourth week he began to have some ability to control his left multifidus using SEMG biofeedback; however, he did not have at that time any sensory awareness of this activation; he relied entirely on the SEMG signal at this point. During the fifth week of rehabilitation it was noted that the patient's left hip flexor strength was improving somewhat. At the same time he began to note the occurrence of sharp, intermittent stabs of pain across the left anterior thigh. His anterior thigh numbness was unchanged. By the eighth week of treatment the patient had good control of a combined transversus and multifidus activation in prone and supine. Prone lying knee flexion, or prone knee bend, was initiated as a limb loading task as prone was the position in which the patient felt most confident in his transversus abdominis and multifidus activation (the prone knee bend is generally more difficult from a motor control perspective than, for example, supine 'bent knee fallouts' and had the potential to tension the femoral nerve; thus, his early response to this exercise was monitored closely).

At ten weeks, the patient's symptoms were notably improved during his ADLs. Repeated testing revealed improved volume of the left multifidus relative to the initial assessment (although still diminished relative to the right side) along with a physiological SLR test. The patient's anterior thigh and knee pain were resolved yet his numbness persisted. He occasionally had some mild soreness over the left PSIS. He was more comfortable in his gait and no longer felt he needed support while descending stairs. He had returned to his job on modified duties - more administrative work than actual auto mechanic work - and was tolerating this well. He was discharged to a home program with instructions to progress his limb loading tasks and to gradually return to his weight training activities in a further four weeks.

Comment:

Certainly this patient was showing signs of improvement on initial assessment. Thus it cannot be stated categorically that this outcome would not have been achieved had it not been for the treatment provided. However the patient did demonstrate objective evidence of neuromuscular improvement (improved skill at activation of transversus and multifidus, decreased atrophy of the lumbar multifidus and a normal SLR test) which coincided in time with his functional and symptomatic improvements.

Case Study 4 (Jemmett)

Subjective Examination:

16 year old female high school student and competitive basketball player. This patient presented with a seven month history of traumatic-onset, bilateral low back pain without symptoms into the lower extremities. Her pain had progressed to the point where she could not play basketball nor participate in physical education classes. She stated that standing was her most uncomfortable position and that her pain was frequently relieved with sitting although she was unable to sit for longer than ten to fifteen minutes without an increase in her low back pain. She had been treatedby a physiotherapist elsewhere for several weeks performing primarily (by the patient's report) stability ball exercises. She denied any history of prior low back pain and stated that her health was otherwise fine.

Objective Examination:

The patient moved cautiously on 'sit to stand' and demonstrated an antalgic gait with a decrease in right stance time. Observation revealed increased tone in the right lumbar and lower thoracic paraspinals. Greater sway along with a slight 'Trendelenburg' sign were evident on the right side with single limb stance testing. AROM was unremarkable through the cardinal planes. However, combined right side flexion with extension elicited her typical low back pain. H & I testing demonstrated a marked loss of extension if right side flexion was the initial movement. A neurogenic Slump test was noted on the right. PIVM testing revealed increased extension at the L4-5 motion segment; the L4-5 SCT demonstrated a notable increase in compliance. Segmental integrity testing (sidelying APSIT) also indicated increased compliance at the L4-5 segment. The L5 and L4 spinous processes were markedly tender on palpation. The multifidus was diminished in volume on the right at L4-5.

Working Diagnosis:

A single level, uni-directional segmental dysfunction or clinical instability involving the L4-5 segment. Any neurodynamic compromise was thought to be relatively minimal.

Prognosis:

This patient's prognosis should have been good to excellent given her examination findings. However, she lived two hours away and could only attend once each week for treatment. The inconvenience of a four-hour round trip and the inability to monitor the patient more regularly were originally seen as factors likely to reduce her chances of attaining an optimal outcome.

Management and Outcome:

The patient's initial treatment session consisted of forty minutes of education with her mother present in addition to ten minutes of IEMS at the right

L4-5 multifidus. As well she was taught a basic pelvic floor - transversus abdominis activation and asked to practice this two to three times daily.

This patient was seen a total of twelve times over a fourteen week period. She was highly motivated despite not being permitted to play basketball at the start of the new school year (six weeks into treatment) and having to drive significant distances for physiotherapy. Following the initial session, treatment consisted only of segmental stabilization exercises. The patient had reasonable control of multifidus in prone and supine following nine weeks of treatment. The patient had a physiological Slump test at this point also. The final three weeks of treatment emphasized a progression to integrated stability ball training. At discharge there was no appreciable loss of multifidus volume at L4-5 (tested *via* palpation). She had demonstrated excellent compliance with her home exercise program and was able to return to all activities without pain approximately four months following her initial session.

Case Study 5 (Jemmett)

Subjective Examination:

52 year old male, married with two children aged 12 and 15. This patient worked as a cable television installer and was otherwise sedentary. His BMI was 29 and he smoked 1/2 pack of cigarettes daily. He stated that he was moderately hypertensive, but well controlled with medication. His previous history included a series of low back pain episodes which he estimated began in his mid-thirties. These episodes lasted up to three weeks although he rarely missed more than a few days work with any single episode. During the more severe episodes he recalled having some leg pain but could not recall which leg was painful.

The patient presented four weeks post-operatively following L4-5 discectomy and five months following the initial onset of back pain. His injury had occurred as he got out of bed one morning; he described his initial symptoms as a 'massive shot of pain from my back to my foot'. He had waited three weeks to see the surgeon, another six to obtain an MRI examination and then another seven weeks prior to having his surgery. During this period he had both low back and right lower extremity pain (lateral right leg and foot) which he described as approximately equal in intensity. He had only been able to tolerate sitting for a maximum of ten minutes and had spent much of the pre-operative period either standing or lying down. He had not worked since the initial onset of his symptoms.

Following his surgery he had been told by his surgeon to engage in light physical activity as tolerated; he had been given the referral to physiotherapy for *muscle strengthening* at his four week surgical follow-up. He was pleased that the majority of his right lower extremity pain had been alleviated with surgery; however, he had persistent lumbar spine pain which he described as a 'throbbing ache' just to the side of his incision along with mild right lower extremity pain with sitting. He was concerned that perhaps the surgeon had missed something given that he still had some back and leg pain. Aggravating factors at four weeks post-surgery included sitting for longer than 15 minutes and bending forward to shave or work at the kitchen counter. He did not think he would be ready to return to his job 'any time soon'.

Objective Examination:

Lumbar AROM was tested in sitting. Sidebending was limited bilaterally to approximately 50% with the patient reporting an increase in his typical low back pain in each direction. Flexion was limited to just less than 25% by the same pain. Combined movement testing was not performed. The seated straight leg raise demonstrated limited knee extension bilaterally (the patient described 'tight' hamstrings) without reproduction of back or thigh pain. The Slump test gave a physiological result on the left side and a neurogenic response on the right. A neurological scan examination revealed an absent achilles reflex on the right side along with marked weakness of the great toe extensors on the right.

PIVM testing demonstrated progressively decreased flexion from the L3-4 to the L5-S1 segment. Indeed, at L5-S1 there was virtually no flexion noted. The flexion SCT at this level was very stiff. However, there was markedly increased compliance or 'give' with the rotary SIT at L4-5. On palpation there appeared to be a bilateral loss of multifidus volume at L4-5 and L5-S1 relative to the upper lumbar spine. He was able to activate his transversus abdominis briefly following several minutes of education however he felt the need to fully activate his pelvic floor in order to get even slight activity in transversus abdominis.

Working Diagnosis:

Post-surgical, multi-directional clinical instability involving the L4-5 motion segment along with a marked hypomobility at L5-S1.

Prognosis:

This patient's prognosis was estimated to be only poor to moderate. A number of factors acted as negative prognostic indicators in this analysis. His general health status was not ideal, he had a lengthy, episodic history of low back pain and several months had elapsed since the initial onset of the severe episode which eventually led to his surgery. A number of architectural changes affecting each of the passive and active subsystems would likely have developed secondary to both the underlying pathology and the surgery itself. Finally, his inability to activate transversus abdominis on initial examination might have suggested a greater than average degree of difficulty in learning the therapeutic exercises. On the positive side of the prognostic ledger, the patient was appreciated to be highly motivated and likely to be to be compliant with his proposed management program.

Treatment Plan and Outcome:

This patient's initial management involved extensive education regarding the nature of his pre and post-surgical dysfunction and the rationale for treatment. The first two treatment sessions included IEMS at the right L4-5 multifidus, facilitation of transversus abdominis and flexion mobilizations at L5-S1. The patient did not realize any significant improvement in range or symptoms following IEMS. Treatment continued, emphasizing differential activation of the transversus abdominis and multifidus muscles from the multi-segmental muscles along with mobilization of the L5-S1 segment.

Following six weeks of treatment averaging one to two sessions per week the patient had very good control of the multifidus in supine with and without SEMG biofeedback. He was able to maintain this activation while performing fourth stage activities in supine such as the bent knee fall-out and the heel slide; however, he was unable to develop good control of the multifidus in prone. His symptoms had been gradually improving throughout treatment and prior to him developing control of transversus abdominis and multifidus. He was discharged at nine weeks with improved sitting tolerances and an ability to do most of the tasks required at his job. Flexion at L5-S1 was somewhat improved and he had maintained good control of transversus abdominis and multifidus in supine. He did not develop control of multifidus in prone by discharge.

Comment:

This patient likely realized some therapeutic success *via* these interventions however it is expected that much of his symptomatic improvement occurred for reasons other than his attendance at physiotherapy. He did not have the typical rapid response to IEMS nor did his change in symptoms strongly coincide with his ability to control his transversus abdominis and multifidus. Indeed, this gentleman continues to have low back pain although his lower extremity symptoms have not bothered him for over two years. As discussed previously, it is likely that our ability to rehabilitate the neural control subsystem and muscles such transversus abdominis and multifidus is to some extent limited, and perhaps by the degree of pathology or dysfunction present at the segment.

Case Study 6 (MacDonald)

Subjective Examination:

A 34 year old female presented to the clinic with a two week history of 'sharp' low back pain along with pain into the right buttock. She described her symptoms as being of gradual onset and non-traumatic in origin. She also complained of numbness along her distal lateral right leg and the dorsum of her right foot. The pain in her low back was described as a 'horrible' kind of pain; the buttock pain was characterized as 'achy'. Aggravating factors included transitional movements such as sit to stand and lying to sitting. She stated that sitting with equal weightbearing through the pelvis increased her right buttock pain. She demonstrated that if she sat with her weight through her left hemipelvis her symptoms decreased (her trunk moved into flexion and left side flexion). Her symptoms had been increasing in the days preceding her initial visit.

Previous medical history included a ten year history of stress incontinence. She reported a recent surgery to correct this problem along with a tubal ligation. Since this surgery she had noted a loss in abdominal muscle 'tone'. She described a history of episodic right foot pain. On direct questioning she denied any history of previous low back pain. She was obese, generally sedentary with no noted form of physical activity, and smoked one to two packs of cigarettes per day. She had one ten year old son and worked full time as an insurance company customer service representative. She had not taken any medication for the symptoms as she "did not like to take pills unless she absolutely had to".

Objective Examination:

Active lumbar movements were assessed in sitting. Left sidebending was unremarkable while right sidebending was limited to 25% of normal and reproduced her typical low back and buttock pain. Combined left sidebending plus flexion was less limited and painful than was flexion alone. When asked to actively extend her lumbar spine, the patient extended her cervical spine only and, not surprisingly, did not report any low back pain; on more directed lumbar extension, the movement was markedly limited and very painful - the patient described this as her 'sharp' low back pain.

The slump test demonstrated a neurogenic response on the right with knee extension limited by 45 degrees; the patient had reproduction of both her lumbar and right buttock pain with this test. On the left, knee extension was full but this elicited some 'pulling' in her low back. The neurological screening examination was unremarkable.

The patient was placed in left side lying (her painful side 'up' - the patient was more comfortable on her left and it gave the clinician improved access to the painful right side). With the patient passively positioned into trunk/hip flexion, provocation of her low back pain was noted at approximately 85 degrees of hip flexion. The patient was maintained in this position, at P1, to perform segmental compliance testing (SCTs). Testing could be performed at P1 of lumbar flexion as the patient was able to fully relax despite mild provocation of symptoms. Cranially directed PA's intended to mimic her limited active flexion range were performed at each lumbar spinous process. The cranially directed PA at the L5 spinous process was described as mildly tender, L4 was very tender and L3 was symptom free. Unfortunately the L4-5 motion segment could not be stressed into resistance with this type of testing, as the patient described such attempts as "too painful". Thus it was not possible to determine the degree of connective tissue 'give' at this segment. However, the fact that this segment was so irritable to mechanical stress while in a flexed position was certainly informative.

With the patient remaining in left side lying, the patient's lumbar spine was moved into a neutral and symptom free position. The sidelying APSIT revealed increased connective tissue give or compliance at L4-5 relative to the L3-4 motion segment. All other integrity testing was unremarkable. There was a significant decrease in muscle bulk of the L4-5 multifidus on the right. The patient demonstrated breath holding, along with co-contraction of her hip adductors and hamstrings when attempting to contract transversus abdominis in supine crook-lying.

Working Diagnosis:

A single-level, uni-directional clinical instability at L4-5 with adverse neurodynamics.

Prognosis:

Although this patient likely had only a single plane instability, her prognosis was considered to be limited, as many other factors could have negatively effected her outcome. She had a long history of stress incontinence in addition to recent pelvic floor reconstruction and abdominal surgery; each of these would have interfered with both her abdominal and pelvic floor muscle function. She was sedentary and in relatively poor health (smoking & obesity). There was also a clear involvement of nervous tissue in her presentation. Her occupation required her to sit for a large percentage of her day, which could have also negatively effected her outcome. For this patient to have been successful she would have had to overcome many obstacles in order to improve the function of her neuromuscular system sufficient to gain control of segmental motion at her L4-5 motion segment. Her expectations of treatment appeared reasonable.

Management and Outcome:

This patient's initial treatment program consisted of considerable education regarding her condition and what would be required of her in order to attain her treatment objectives. Her previous medical history and its negative influences on both her current status and her ability to fully control her symptoms were also explained. The patient was instructed to activate her transversus abdominis in left side lying as this was her most comfortable position. In addition, IEMS was utilized at the dysfunctional segment of multifidus muscle at the right L4-5 motion segment. Immediately following this treatment session she demonstrated a 50% improvement in active right side bending along with a significant increase in the amount of knee extension available on the right with repeated Slump testing. She was advised to limit her static sitting to no longer than fifteen minutes at a time if at all possible.

At the second visit she described a period of symptom relief following the initial visit. She did state that her usual symptoms had since returned. She stated that she was not sure that she was performing her abdominal exercise properly. Her lumbar AROM was similar to that seen on initial examination. The patient was treated in a similar fashion during the second visit. The emphasis of treatment during that visit was on the differential activation of transversus abdominis and the patient's awareness of this muscle. Similar improvement was seen after this visit. At this point the patient was informed that her symptoms would likely continue to return as she was not yet able to integrate this enhanced coordination of the segmental stabilizing muscles into functional activities. As a result she was unable to support and control motion at the dysfunctional segment.

She was seen intermittently over a period of eight weeks for a total of six visits. She noticed an increase in her awareness of the transversus abdominis and multifidus muscles. She was able to easily co-contract these muscles in non-weightbearing positions and she progressed to stage four of the therapeutic exercise program. However, she continued to have some difficulty maintaining this co-contraction in static weight-bearing positions. She had noticed an ability to control her symptoms with a voluntary activation of the segmental stabilizing muscles during activities of daily living. Her AROM in sitting was full and symptom-free when she was last seen. Her Slump test revealed only physiological responses to stretch. She was asked to continue with her home exercise program of transversus abdominis & multifidus co-contraction in crook-lying and to attempt to initiate lower limb movement as able. This was considered a reasonable outcome given the patient's initial examination findings.

Case Study 7 (MacDonald)

Subjective Examination:

A 51 year old male presented to the clinic with a one month history of gradually increasing non-traumatic, right-sided buttock, medial knee and lateral anklc pain. These symptoms were described as intermittent but 'sharp'. The patient also noted that his symptomatic right leg felt shorter than the left. Walking and climbing stairs were consistently provocative of his symptoms. As a result he was unable to walk for any distance without having to stop due to pain. Otherwise his medical and social histories were unremarkable. He had used NSAID's but they had no appreciable effect on his symptoms. He worked as an administrator and normally exercised three times per week; he had been unable to train in recent weeks secondary to his symptoms.

Objective Examination:

Observation of gait demonstrated decreased right hip extension during late stance and decreased stride length; the amount of time spent in the stance phase was symmetrical. The lower thoracic spine appeared slightly kyphotic in standing. While active lumbar movements were limited into flexion by 25 to 50% this was not especially provocative; the patient was limited more by a feeling of 'tightness' in the posterior thigh than by low back or lower extremity pain. Extension was 50% and the patient described a feeling of dull, 'pressure-ish' pain in the lower right lumbar spine. Although the lower lumbar spine extended, the upper lumbar and lower thoracic regions remained kyphotic. The combined movement of right side bending and extension was limited to 50% reproducing the patient's lumbar and right buttock pain. The combined movements of right side bending and flexion were limited to 50% but were non-painful.

The Slump test demonstrated a clinical response - a slight loss of range on the right side with a feeling of 'tightness' into the posterolateral thigh and leg rather than the patient's typical pain. The tightness was reduced with cervical extension. Sensitizing additions to the slump test did not produce a neurogenic response. A neurological screening examination was unremarkable. PIVM testing revealed excessive movement into extension at L4-5 relative to adjacent segments. There was also a decreased amount of flexion at that segment. Segmental compliance testing using a cranially directed PA at the L5 spinous process at R1 of extension revealed excessive connective tissue give at the L4-5 motion segment. A cranially directed PA at the L4 spinous process at R1 of flexion of the L4-5 motion segment demonstrated decreased connective tissue give or compliance. Segmental integrity testing was unremarkable. Examination of the thoracolumbar region revealed a loss of extension and right sidebending at the T10-11 motion segment.

Passive examination of the hip joint demonstrated a firm capsular end feel with marked limitation of hip flexion at only 85 degrees. An attempt to flex and adduct the hip resulted in groin pain. Hip extension was limited to approximately 10 degrees of hip flexion with a firm capsular end feel.

Palpation of the lumbar multifidus revealed segmental loss of muscle bulk at the L4-5 level on the right. The patient was not able to appropriately activate the transversus abdominis. The patient excessively contracted the oblique abdominals and was not able to maintain a normal breathing pattern when attempting to contract transversus abdominis in supine crook-lying.

Working Diagnosis:

This patient developed what could best be described as an extension dysfunction at L4-5 compounded by a lack of hip and upper lumbar extension. It was hypothesized that his lower lumbar spine was forced into a compressive extension pattern during gait resulting in his symptoms. While the findings of reduced L4-5 flexion and a 'normal' segmental integrity test might dissuade us from describing this as a clinical instability, the fact that the L4-5 right multifidus was diminished in bulk suggests that there was dysfunction of both the active and neural control subsystems. Clinically, this must be addressed. His faulty active and neural control subsystem were likely failing to provide adequate control of motion at the L4-5 motion segment as it moved into extension.

Prognosis:

This patient's prognosis was generally good because of his health status; however, the loss of motion above and below the dysfunctional segment did make it difficult for him to avoid aggravating his dysfunction during daily activities. It was suspected that significant degenerative changes at the hip were the cause of the hip hypomobility (this was later confirmed by radiographic examination). It was anticipated that the extent to which the patient's hip movement could be improved would be an important factor in the patient's ability to attain his therapeutic goals. It was reasonable for the patient to presume that he would be able to return to his previous level of activity given his history.

Management and Outcome:

This patient's treatment program focused on improving flexion and left sidebending at the right L4-5 motion segment using a direct flexion technique and extension at the right T10-11 using an indirect extension technique. Restoration of hip extension was also attempted *via* passive hip extension mobilization with the patient in prone with pillows under the patient's abdomen to prevent the lumbar spine from moving into extension. IEMS was utilized at the right L4-5 multifidus. A rehabilitation program for the segmental stabilizing muscles was also initiated. This patient was seen over a six week period for a total of twelve visits. His ability to co-contract transversus abdominis and multifidus while adding lower limb load was achieved within four weeks. Some improvement was made in the lower thoracic spine extension and right sidebending as well as in flexion and left sidebending at the right L4-5

motion segment. However, despite our best clinical efforts, the patient's hip extension was not significantly improved.

Functionally, the patient was able to return to walking to work but any increase in his activity such as ice hockey increased his symptoms. He was discharged with a home program to maintain his lumbar AROM and his muscle function as able.

Case Study 8 (MacDonald)

Subjective Examination:

A 30 year old female presented to the clinic with a three day history of sudden onset right sided low back pain which was present upon waking in the morning. She could not recall any trauma nor significant changes in her activities which could account for these symptoms. She described her pain as 'sharp' and her back as feeling like it was going to 'snap off' if she bent forward. Any quick movement was also painful. She had tried to manage her symptoms by minimizing her physical activity and with massage therapy. To date, her symptoms had remained unchanged. She worked as a window designer, a job requiring heavy lifting, stressful deadlines and long hours. She played soccer and ice hockey and trained (both aerobic and strength training) three days per week. She had no children. Her medical history was otherwise unremarkable with no previous history of low back pain and she was not currently taking any medications. The patient expected that she would fully recover.

Objective Examination:

On observation, the patient's standing posture was unremarkable. Lumbar AROM was assessed in standing. Extension was limited to 25% and reproduced the patient's sharp low back pain. Right side bending was limited to 50%, again reproducing her right sided low back pain. Flexion was limited to less than 50% and also reproduced the patient's right sided back pain. Combined movements were not tested given the extent of the patient's symptoms on cardinal plane testing. The Slump test demonstrated a neurogenic response, i.e., the test elicited low back pain with right knee extension; cervical extension decreased this pain. A neurological scanning examination was unremarkable.

PIVM testing revealed an excessive amount of extension at the L4-5 motion segment. At the patient's limit of L4-5 extension, segmental compliance testing (a cranially directed PA at the L5 spinous process) reproduced her typical low back pain; increased connective tissue compliance or 'give' was also noted at this segment. There was a decreased amount of flexion at the L3-4 motion segment with decreased compliance or 'give' noted with a cranially directed PA at the L3 spinous process. The sidelying APSIT at the L4-5 motion segment revealed an increase in connective tissue compliance. On palpation there was evidence of decreased muscle bulk of the right L4-5 multifidus. She was able to achieve an independent contraction of transversus abdominis with some instruction and verbal feedback.

Working Diagnosis:

This patient presented with a single level, uni-directional clinical instability at the L4-5 motion segment. The loss of motion at the L3-4 segment into flexion might have been a contributing factor as it could prevent the patient's L4-5 segment from moving out of the painful position of extension. There was evidence of neural tissue involvement as evidenced by the Slump test findings.

Prognosis:

This patient was thought to have a good to excellent prognosis. She was otherwise healthy, fit and she was highly motivated. She had a single level, uni-directional dysfunction and reasonably good motor control abilities. Her expectations of treatment were reasonable.

Management and Outcome:

Immediately following the initial assessment, the patient was treated with spinal manipulation into flexion at the L3-4 motion segment along with IEMS at the right L4-5 motion segment. Post-treatment, the patient's flexion was improved to 75 percent of normal with no sensation of pain. The slump test was also improved in that while knee extension remained somewhat reduced, the patient's back pain was no longer reproduced.

Over the next two weeks the patient was instructed to co-contract the transversus abdominis and multifidus muscles and had progressed to the third stage exercises. At this point her symptoms were well controlled and she returned to all physical activities. Given the patient's activity level, it was recommended that she continue and progress through to the fifth stage exercise skills; however, she declined and was thus discharged.

Case Study 9 (MacDonald)

Subjective Examination:

A 31 year old male presented to the clinic describing a six month history of insidious onset, episodic and progressive low back pain. He noted that the frequency of his episodes had been increasing and that he was now experiencing pain 'shooting' into the left lower extremity. On specific questioning, he denied any history of paraesthesia of any kind into the lower extremity. Aggravating factors included any form of lifting, static sitting and bending forward. Despite this history, he was asymptomatic at the time of the initial evaluation. He was married with two young children. He was a self-employed small business owner and reported a very busy schedule given his work and family demands. He stated that he worked out with weights three times per week and that typically his symptoms improved following a workout. He had been prescribed muscle relaxants and NSAIDs, neither of which had any impact on his symptoms. With the exception of his low back pain he was otherwise healthy and had no significant medical history. The patient was highly motivated and keen to return to his normal activities as soon as possible.

Objective Examination:

The patient appeared fit with an athletic build. In standing, there appeared to be a marked increase in muscle tone throughout the left paraspinals. The lumbar spine appeared to be maintained in an extended position from L4 superiorly. Below this level the spine was clearly flexed. There was a lateral deviation to the right along with visible effusion at the L5 spinal level.

Active lumbar range assessed in standing revealed flexion to be only 25%; this was limited by the patient's typical low back pain and a 'pulling' sensation into the left lower extremity. Active extension in the lumbar spine was essentially nil. Right sidebending was limited to 50% by pain and a pulling sensation at the left lumbar region. Left sidebending was essentially nil. Combined movements were not tested given the degree of symptoms reproduced with cardinal plane testing.

The Slump test revealed extremely limited knee extension on the right; the patient was unable to extend the knee beyond 80 degrees of flexion. This increased the patient's typical low back pain along with the lower extremity pain. A neurological screening examination revealed a diminished S1 reflex on the left.

PIVM testing demonstrated a gross loss of extension at the L5-S1 motion segment with a firm end feel. This did not reproduce the patient's symptoms significantly. The L5-S1 segment seem-ed fixed in flexion. The L4-5 motion segment demonstrated a marked lack of flexion; indeed, it was difficult to appreciate any amount of flexion at this segment. However, there was excessive extension present at L4-5. Segmental compliance testing (a cranially directed PA at the L5 spinous process) revealed excessive connective tissue give and reproduced the patient's low back pain.

Segmental integrity testing revealed extreme connective tissue laxity at the L5-S1 mobile segment. It seemed that there was actually palpable movement of L5 on S1 with this test. However,

this test did not reproduce the patient's symptoms. A rotational segmental integrity test also revealed excessive connective tissue give or compliance at L5-S1. No increase in compliance was noted with similar tests at L4-5. On palpation there was marked segmental atrophy of the lumbar multifidus at the L5-S1 level bilaterally. No palpable contraction of the transversus abdominis could be elicited during the initial examination.

Working Diagnosis:

A multi-planar segmental instability at the L5-S1 motion segment with nerve root compromise. The generalized hypomobility with active movement of the lumbar spine was interpreted as being the result of an antalgic posture which had been assumed in order to achieve some degree of control or immobilization over this severe segmental instability. The neural finding, i.e., the diminished S1 reflex, was suggestive of not just nerve tissue irritation, but true compromise. It was assumed that any symptom relief the patient had experienced with exercise was due to pain modulation *via* mechanoreceptor input and perhaps an increase in fluidity of any inflammatory exudates which may have been present.

Prognosis:

This patient was thought to have a poor prognosis. He presented with a progressive history, a multi-directional clinical instability and evidence of nerve root compromise. Unfortunately, this patient's expectation of treatment (a relatively quick return to normal physical activities) was likely unreasonable.

Management and Outcome:

A great deal of time was spent in educating the patient with regard to the examination findings and of his prognosis with conservative management. The patient was treated with exercises to improve the function of the segmental stabilizing muscles. The patient made no significant progress with his therapeutic exercise program or with his symptoms. He was referred at that time to a colleague for evaluation however no new findings or treatment recommendations were forthcoming. The patient was discharged at this time.

On follow up several weeks later the patient's symptoms had continued to increase and he was scheduled for consultation with an orthopaedic surgeon to discuss surgical options.

Case Study 10 (MacDonald)

Subjective Examination:

A 47 year old female presented to the clinic with an eight week history of insidious onset right foot pain, typically felt in the distal plantar aspect of her foot with occasional pain into the heel. She described her symptoms as intense and achy. Typically her symptoms were minimal in the morning. Her pain was aggravated by walking and prolonged standing; her pain was usually worse if she felt tired at the end of a long day. She stated that a hot bath often relieved her foot pain. She worked as an office worker and was generally active exercising three times per week (fitness program and belly dancing).

In recent weeks her foot pain had become worse and she had been unable to manage her pain. She had given up her exercise program due to her symptoms. She had seen her family physician and was diagnosed as having a 'flexor tendonitis'. Prescription NSAIDs had not decreased her symptoms. She was then referred for physiotherapy. The patient's medical history was unremarkable with the exception of episodic low back pain which was not bothering her at the time of her initial examination. Her goal of treatment was to decrease her symptoms so that she could return to her fitness program and belly dancing.

Objective Examination:

On examination, an effusion at the plantar aspect of the forefoot near the second metatarsal was noted. The plantar aspect of the forefoot was significantly tender on palpation. Altered sensation (light touch) at the dorsum of the right foot was noted in comparison to the left. Active and passive testing of the ankle, subtalar and forefoot failed to demonstrate any abnormality in movement. Resisted testing of the long flexors of the foot was unremarkable. The only means of reproducing her symptoms at this point was *via* palpation.

Based on the lack of findings indicative of local pathology, the tenderness on palpation and the altered sensation, a Slump test was performed. The Slump test was modified so as to develop maximum tensioning of the nerves which travel through the plantar and medial aspect of the foot. The ankle was dorsiflexed and the subtalar joint everted prior to the other components of the test. This modified Slump test revealed both a gross loss of knee extension and a mild amount of plantar foot pain. The examination was conducted in the morning when the patient's symptoms generally were less severe; one would thus anticipate having greater difficulty reproducing her symptoms at this time of day.

Given the patient's history and the positive Slump test, a lumbar examination was performed. Standing AROM was reduced by 25% into combined extension and right sidebending. This test reproduced the patient's typical low back pain. Combined flexion and left sidebending was reduced by 50% by a significant feeling of tension in the posterior right thigh. PIVM testing demonstrated a loss of flexion at both the L5-S1 and L4-5 motion segments. Passive extension was not limited in the lumbar spine; however, overpressure of L5-S1 into extension created some local pain. The sidelying APSIT revealed an excess amount of connective tissue give at L5-S1. Decreased multifidus bulk was noted at L5-S1 on the right.

A further modification of the slump test was then performed in left side-lying. The patient's trunk was flexed along with her cervical spine. The patient was then asked to extend her right knee. With application of a PIVM into combined flexion and left sidebending, the patient reported an increase in posterior thigh tension. With a maintained PIVM, decreased knee extension was available when in the Slump position, i.e., in a position of neural tension vs. non-neural tension. The neurological screening examination was unremarkable.

Working Diagnosis:

This patient presented with an L5-S1 clinical instability and associated adverse neurodynamics. The pain at the plantar-aspect of the right foot, the swelling and sensory changes at the dorsum of the foot were, in this case, not representative of peripheral pathology. These were manifestations of peripheral nervous tissue irritation secondary to the clinical instability in the lumbar spine.

Prognosis:

As the patient was otherwise in good health and presented with only a uni-planar instability it was expected that she would recover although this would likely be a slow process given the degree of neural involvement. Her expectations of treatment were certainly reasonable.

Management and Outcome:

This patient was treated with IEMS at the right L4-5 multifidus, manipulation into flexion at L4-5 and a program of segmental stability exercises. The manipulation was intended to facilitate the patient's ability to move out of the extended position at this segment, a finding which was interpreted as perpetuating her symptoms.

Following ten sessions over a two month period, the patient demonstrated an improved ability to control her segmental stabilizing muscles under load in both static and dynamic conditions. Lumbar flexion was improved as was her Slump test. The inflammation and paraesthesia at the right forefoot also resolved. The patient reported a significant decrease in her symptoms and was able to return to her physical activities. She was advised to continue with her therapeutic exercise program to ensure a full recovery and maintain control of her symptoms.

CHAPTER **EIGHT**

invited commentary

The peer reviewed literature often utilizes the 'invited commentary' as a means of providing a considered, expert perspective on a novel or controversial concept. An example is Martin Krag's commentary on Panjabi's neutral zone and stabilization systems papers of 1992. Such commentaries may support or challenge the findings or interpretations set forth in the original article. Regardless of whether a commentary reflects positively or negatively on the primary article, it should certainly inspire further debate and consideration. Our objectives for this final chapter were to help foster a necessary transparency within the physiotherapy textbook literature and hopefully present a variety of perspectives on the potential clinical significance of our text, the current clinically relevant evidence, and, in general, the management of lumbar pathology by physiotherapy clinicians.

Following completion of this text, the authors contacted twelve individuals considered experts in the areas of either orthopaedic clinical practice, neuromusculoskeletal research, physiotherapy education and/or evidence-based practice. These individuals lived and worked in either the United Kingdom, Canada, the United States or Australia. The authors had pre-existing professional relationships with two of the twelve people invited to comment on the text. The candidates were asked if they would be willing to read the final draft of the text, and provide an objective and balanced critique. The authors agreed that as many as five commentaries would be published, with the selection decision based solely on a first-to-accept basis. The candidates were not informed as to the identity of the other contributors until after all submissions were received.

We would like to extend our sincere appreciation to the four individuals who accepted this invitation. In alphabetical order, they are:

- Susan R Harris, PhD, PT
- Peter Huijbregts, PT, MSc, MHSc, DPT
- Robert Johnson, PT, MS
- Shaun Lapenskie, M.Manip. PT, BSc (PT)

Each agreed to work under a restrictive timeline and therefore needed to shuffle existing priorities and commitments in order to meet our publication deadline. We thank them all for their insight and enthusiasm, and their willingness to be a part of this project.

RJ & DM

Susan R Harris PhD, PT, FAPTA

Susan Harris is a professor in the School of Rehabilitation Sciences, University of British Columbia and an associate member of the Department of Pediatrics at the Children's & Women's Health Centre of British Columbia. She is also the Scientific Editor of the peer-reviewed journal *Physiotherapy Canada*. Dr. Harris' research interests include the early diagnosis of cerebral palsy and the effects of exercise on women living with breast cancer. Dr. Harris also has a keen interest in evidence-based medicine and the interactions between health care professionals and their patients.

As a long-time pediatric physiotherapist who has dabbled more recently in breast cancer rehabilitation research, you can imagine my surprise when one of the authors of *Physiotherapeutic Management of Lumbar Spine Pathology* invited me to write a commentary on this book. As someone whose physiotherapy training pre-dated any education in orthopedic manual therapy, what could I possibly contribute?

In his kind invitation to review this book and write a commentary, Rick Jemmett assured me that he and David MacDonald were far more interested in my viewpoint as a longstanding and vocal proponent of evidence-based practice than in my rudimentary (and seriously outdated) orthopedic skills. I breathed a big sigh of relief and decided to tackle this interesting project head on!

According to Sackett and colleagues (2000), evidence-based medicine has been defined as: "The conscientious, explicit and judicious use of current best evidence in making decisions about the care of individual patients. EBM is the integration of "best research evidence with clinical expertise and patient values." In the book's Introduction, the authors state that their primary objective is "to develop and present a clinical model of lumbar spine pathology which is both evidence-based and clinically relevant." The authors are to be congratulated for including recent, primary research references to substantiate many of their clinically based comments and suppositions, particularly in chapters 1 – 4. Unfortunately, there was far less research evidence to support the information provided in the latter three chapters that comprise the most important part of the book (assessment, management, and clinical case studies).

Many of the authors' suggested assessment and intervention strategies were unsubstantiated by recent research evidence.

The third element of Sackett and colleagues' definition of evidence-based practice, the integration of patient values, is not as apparent in the book. In chapter 1, *Towards a New Paradigm in Patient Management*, the inclusion of the patient's values as one of the foundations of the Segmental Dysfunction Model would have made this model a refreshing and truly 'new' paradigm. Instead, it is a deficit or dysfunction-oriented model, rather than a model that successfully incorporates all three components of evidence-based practice.

While it is laudable in any new book to include clinical case studies (chapter 7), there was inconsistent reference to patients' involvement in determining their own assessment and management plans. Although a global 'goals statement' was included in the introduction to this chapter, the individual case studies (and the clients themselves) would have benefited from the inclusion of individual, measurable therapy objectives that were developed collaboratively by the client and the practitioner (Randall & McEwen, 2000). One good example in which this did occur was in the first case study in which the patient's goal was to run a half-marathon without knee pain. This represents an objective and measurable client-centered goal. Research involving physicians and their patients has shown that patients who were more informed and more involved in their own decision-making were not only more accepting of their treatment regimens but also experienced better health outcomes

(Simpson et al., 1991; Stewart et al., 1999).

In addition to the authors' inconsistent inclusion of measurable, collaborative, client-centered objectives for assessment and treatment in the clinical case studies, I found that many of the statements made were vague and subjective, especially those involving diagnosis, prognosis, and patient change. Diagnostic terms such as "mild segmental dysfunction", "increased tone", and "inappropriate patterning" are entirely subjective. None of these terms are actually measurable (nor were they measured). Many terms used in the "objective examination" sections also failed to be objective and, although some were actually measurable, no measurements were provided, e.g. "increased lumbar lordosis", "marked contraction", "significantly lower degree of (muscle) activity". Objective examination terms, such as "marked weakness" and "reduced stance time", could easily have been measured by a manual muscle test and a stopwatch, respectively. The lack of true measurements during supposedly "objective" examinations represents a serious shortcoming in these patient vignettes and eliminates the opportunity to note objective change as a result of interventions.

Prognostic terminology was particularly subjective, e.g. "poor to moderate", "good to excellent". What do these terms actually mean? Would two therapists be able to agree on these prognoses given that none of these terms has been operationally defined? Wouldn't the therapist's clinical reasoning (see chapter 4) be enhanced by prognostic categories that are well defined, mutually exclusive, exhaustive and measurable? Operationally defining and measuring patient outcomes or projecting prognoses is also central to evidence-based practice. This is something I learned more than 25 years ago in my graduate education and yet this concept has yet to be embraced by most practicing clinicians.

The sub-title to this book is "An evidence-based, best practice clinical model incorporating prospective clinical reasoning, manual therapy, and segmental stabilization exercises." To me, best practice incorporates informed, shared decision-making with clients as well as individualized, measurable client-centered therapy objectives to assess the success (or lack thereof) of the interventions we provide. As well, an evidence-based model should incorporate patient values along with the best research evidence and clinical expertise. The authors have included 'patient values' in at least three of the case examples and for this they are to be congratulated.

The authors have done an admirable job of approaching a difficult task and I am grateful to them for inviting me to write this commentary. I hope that subsequent editions of this book will more fully incorporate the 'patient voice' in clinical decision-making and will truly facilitate the best practice of orthopedic physiotherapists by consistently modeling the use of measurable client-centered goals and outcomes with well-defined, objective terminology.

References

Randall KE, McEwen IR. Writing patient-centered functional goals. Phys Ther 2000;80:1197-1203.

Sackett DL, Strauss SE, Richardson WS., et al. *Evidence-Based Medicine: How to Practice and Teach EBM*, 2nd Ed. 2000 New York: Churchill Livingstone.

Simpson M, Buckman R, Stewart M, Magyar P, Lipkin M, Novak D, Till J. Doctor-patient communication: the Toronto consensus statement. BMJ 1991;303:1385-1387.

Stewart M, Brown JB, Boon H, Galajda J, Meredith L, Sangster M. Evidence on patient-doctor communication. Cancer Prev Con 1999;3:25-30.

Peter Huijbregts, PT, MSc, MHSc, DPT, FAAOMPT, FCAMT

Peter Huijbregts is a clinical physiotherapist in private practice in Victoria, British Columbia. He is also an assistant professor of online education with the University of St. Augustine for Health Sciences. Recently, Peter became the Editor of the *Journal of Manual and Manipulative Therapy* after serving as its associate editor for five years. He is also a reviewer for a number of other peer-reviewed journals including *Physical Therapy* and *Physiotherapy Canada*. His own educational history spans two continents and five countries. He has published extensively on a variety of topics related to orthopaedic manual therapy, including lumbar spine pathology and evidence-based practice. He has provided continuing education programs for clinicians in The Netherlands and throughout the United States.

When I first received the manuscript for this book, the subtitle immediately caught my attention. Providing an evidence-based, best-practice clinical model for physiotherapeutic management of lumbar spine dysfunction seemed like an extremely worthwhile, yet hard to achieve goal. The paradigm of evidence-based practice (EBP) pervades all aspects of modern medicine; physiotherapy is not and should not be an exception[1]. EBP has been defined as the process of integrating the best research evidence available with both clinical expertise and patients' values[2]. As such, this new paradigm represented a significant shift away from the traditional physiotherapy paradigm, which relied heavily on a pathophysiologic and pathobiomechanical rationale. However, there are substantial criticisms to EBP. Most relevant to the topic of lumbar spine dysfunction is the fact that, despite a growing body of research evidence in this area, frequently no relevant direct evidence exists from basic or applied research to answer a specific clinical question. Pathophysiologic and pathobiomechanical rationale are still required to provide direction for patient management and when integrated with the EBP paradigm they provide a best-practice clinical model.

In this book, the authors present the segmental dysfunction model as a basis for evaluation and management of patients with lumbar spine dysfunction. Rather than attempting to isolate a particular pathological structure or overemphasizing psychosocial dimensions of the health problem the authors hypothesize that a decrease in segmental stiffness along with altered activity in segmental and multi-segmental muscles is the prominent dysfunction in patients previously diagnosed with non-specific low back pain (LBP). Based on this hypothesis they have constructed an extremely logical and practical approach to evaluation and management of patients with LBP with an emphasis on identifying and restoring adequate segmental motion and motor control.

The authors provide a thorough review of the available evidence on lumbar spine dysfunction covering histological, electrophysiological, biomechanical, and clinical outcome studies relevant to the topic. They combine this research-based information with a discussion of anatomy, proposed pathobiomechanics and pathophysiology, and relevant manual therapy examination techniques thus producing the best-practice clinical model mentioned in the subtitle.

Of course, the pathobiomechanical and pathophysiologic components of the segmental dysfunction model require further study. As of yet, there is limited or no evidence for the reliability and validity of the manual therapy examination techniques described in this book[3-5]. The clinical outcome studies referenced in this book certainly do not prove the theories on the role of segmental motor control beyond a doubt. However, in my opinion the authors are to be commended for providing a logical and clinically very useful analysis and interpretation of relevant literature. My personal clinical practice, for one, has been impacted positively by reading this book. The authors are also to be commended for setting out to actively answer some of the research questions on this topic in need of answers[6,7]. The Institute of Medicine defined quality of care as the degree to which health care services for individuals and populations increase the likelihood of desired health outcomes and are consistent with current professional knowledge[8]. In my opinion, the authors have certainly succeeded in producing a book that will likely improve the quality of physiotherapeutic care for patients with lumbar spine dysfunction.

References

1. Huijbregts PA. Evidence-based practice. *Interdivisional Review* 2005:Jan/Feb:3.

2. Sackett DL, et al. *Evidence-Based Medicine: How To Practice & Teach EBM*. New York, NY: Churchill Livingstone, 1997.

3. Huijbregts PA. Spinal motion palpation: A review of reliability studies. *J Manual Manipulative Ther* 2002;10:24-39

4. Najm WI, Seffinger MA, Mishra SI, et al. Content validity of manual spinal palpatory exams: A systematic review. *BMC Complementary and Alternative Medicine* 2003;3:1. Available at: http://www.biomedcentral.com/1472-6882/3/1. Accessed March 11, 2005.

5. Tilscher H, Hanna M, Graf E. Klinische und roentgenologische Befunde bei der Hypermobilitaet und Instabilitaet im Lendenwirbelsaeulenbereich. *Manuelle Medizin* 1994;32:1-7.

6. Jemmett RS, MacDonald DA, Agur AMR. Anatomical relationships between selected segmental muscles of the lumbar spine in the context of multi-planar segmental motion: A preliminary investigation. *Man Ther* 2004:9:203-210.

7. MacDonald DA, Hodges PW, Moseley L. The function of the lumbar multifidus in unilateral low back pain. In: *Proceedings of the Fifth Interdisciplinary World Congress on Low Back and Pelvic Pain*. Melbourne, Australia, 2004.

8. Lohr KN, Ed. *Medicare: A Strategy for Quality Assurance*. Washington, DC: National Academy Press, 1990: 21.

Robert Johnson, MSc, PT

Robert Johnson is the owner and clinical director of the *Northwestern Rehabilitation Institute*, and Chair of the American Physical Therapy Association's *Orthopedic Specialty Council*. Robert teaches in the United States and Canada with the NOI Group. Robert has held professional appointments including selection as a Subject Matter Expert (1 of 12 in the US), by the American Board of Physical Therapy Specialties, Orthopedic Section - Task Force on Orthopedic Specialists Examination. In addition to his professional association with the APTA Orthopedic Section, he has most recently held positions as Orthopedic Clinical Specialist with the *Chicago Institute of Neurosurgery & Neuroresearch* and Adjunct Clinical Instructor with the Northwestern University Medical School.

———————————

Current clinical approaches directed towards the physiotherapeutic management of lumbar spine dysfunction are broad and multi-faceted, drawing on information from diverse fields such as biomechanics, physiology, genetics, motor control, pain science, psychology and ergonomics. Our understanding of the variety of clinical patterns that can be present within the realm of 'lumbar dysfunction' continues to develop as clinical research in these fields progresses, and yet a clearly defined path for managing these patients remains elusive.

Clinical application of current evidence-based practice strongly supports manual therapeutic interventions and exercise as key components in positive treatment outcomes for many neuro-musculoskeletal movement dysfunctions. The use of a motor control paradigm as a focus of the exercise component in spinal rehabilitation is not new. The importance of motor control continues to gain significant support from basic science research and clinical trials. This must be considered by clinicians who are committed to using the best available evidence within a clinical reasoning framework towards patient care. MacDonald and Jemmett are to be commended for their timely contribution, interpretations and unique insights regarding the examination and recommended clinical management of this difficult patient population.

Traditional manual therapy models have typically embraced the concept of segmental spinal mobility as either normal, stiff (hypomobile) or excessive (hypermobile). Historically, the emphasis of manual therapy intervention has been directed towards facilitating increased motion to the stiff, hypomobile segment with little regard for those motion segments that seemingly moved too much. This overemphasis in 'finding and fixing' the hypomobile regions may have limited clinical success and weakened treatment outcomes. Interestingly, in some manual therapy approaches the pendulum seems to be swinging away from the 'hypomobility' focus towards the hypermobility (instability) end of the movement spectrum. Let us be aware of past mistakes as we gain further insight in understanding motion and how to treat it clinically. Do not forego recognition of stiffness as a contributing factor in lumbar movement dysfunction and yet allow for it's counterpart, instability, to become a clearer component of clinical presentation than it may have been in the past.

Recognition that mobility is quite variable between individual spinal segments across patient populations is well accepted. However, as clinical emphasis shifts, and as research details a better understanding of the changes that are associated with those segments that may move more significantly, confusion has arisen in trying to define 'instability' in universally acceptable language. MacDonald and Jemmett have done us all a favor in summarizing this body of knowledge and proposing a clinical model of instability useful for further dialogue, debate and application. It is clear that segmental motor control changes occur with lumbar pathology and that elements related to segmental stiffness/compliance are associated with some of these changes. It is necessary therefore to provide treatment interventions directed to enhancing specific segmental motor control as part of a comprehensive evidence based protocol. The motor control applications proposed by the authors are grounded in strong theoretical, basic science and clinical research. Cautious optimism regarding the potential success of this approach within the larger framework of lumbar spine dysfunction is warranted. The unique addition of their case studies, formatted to clearly present subjective/objective findings, supported working diagnosis, prognosis rationale and management/outcome is a benefit to novice clinicians and those less familiar with manual therapy and motor control principles.

However, colleagues who truly embrace a clinical reasoning approach to patient care would be remiss if they were to focus only upon potential instability as the primary approach to the challenges of lumbar spine dysfunction. Evidence within the burgeoning field of pain science is forcing many clinicians to rethink traditional models of pathology and patient presentation in order to incorporate central nervous system mechanisms within the larger framework of movement dysfunction, including lumbar pain pathologies. Our understanding of sensory input mechanisms, central processing states and altered output patterns continue to refine our understand-

ing of the individual, patterns of pain presentation and motor control within this specific population. Allowance for 'the brain' to become a primary player in peripheral/spinal joint dysfunctions, and the manifestations thereof, is a significant movement containing strong evidence that clinicians must embrace and integrate into existing clinical models of care if the science and art of Physical Therapy are to continue.

MacDonald and Jemmett have produced an important piece of clinically relevant material directed towards a difficult patient population. Their thorough review of this literature has allowed them to strongly propose an evidence based examination and patient management guide for lumbar instability. It is a worthy effort and yet it remains a small piece in a seemingly large puzzle. Let us embrace this approach skeptically and with an open mind, not forgetting the traditional methods of manual therapy and exercise which carried us this far, nor the continuing evolution of research that together broadens our clinical reasoning capabilities and contributes to the base of evidence necessary to further enhance positive patient outcomes. The work of MacDonald and Jemmett will be time tested and surely revised, as all good models are, but it is a necessary contribution to our profession and for that we are grateful.

Shaun Lapenskie, BSc, M.Manip. PT (Aus), FCAMT

Shaun Lapenskie obtained his undergraduate physiotherapy degree from the University of Western Ontario in 1997 and in 2000 completed a Masters degree at Curtin University in Perth, Western Australia specializing in the treatment of spinal and musculoskeletal disorders. He presented his graduate research at the World Congress on Low Back Pain in Montreal (2001). He currently serves as co-editor of the *Orthopaedic Division Review*. Central to his treatment philosophy is the idea that manual therapy is nothing without motor control, and that 'hands-on' treatment can only be an adjunct to retraining dysfunctional motor control patterns.

It is perhaps fitting that a clinical perspective comes at the end, as in the end it is with the clinician that 'the rubber meets the road', and dealing with low back pain becomes less of an academic concept and more of a pressing concern. "Theory can leave questions unanswered, but practice has to come up with something", so it is left to clinicians to reconcile current literature to formal education and clinical experience, and develop effective treatment methods. Unfortunately, individual patients tend to not fit easily into textbook definitions of lumbar dysfunction and bring with them unique histories, personalities, and views on how their pain should be addressed.

The enigma of low back pain has been made a great deal clearer with the publication of *Physiotherapeutic Management of Lumbar Spine Pathology*. David MacDonald and Rick Jemmett have assembled a view of the scientific literature that manages to strip away the layers of conjecture and academic argument that frequently cloud the task of treating low back pain, and the result is the Segmental Dysfuntion Model (SDM). The strongest aspect of this model is that it is simple (if any model dealing with lumbar spine dysfunction can be said to be so); to wit: regardless of the pathoanatomy, specific deficits in neuromuscular control tend to develop at the affected segment of the spine; therefore, any treatment must include an attempt to address these deficits to be successful in the long term.

The clinical model is evidence-based and clearly formulated. The review of the literature is compre-

hensive, and the quality of the research cited is, in my opinion, excellent. Clinicians can be assured that the scientific basis for this model is solid.

The assessment and treatment of segmental dysfunction is clearly described and the authors' focus on learning low-level tasks before progressing to higher-level tasks is important to note. One must not try to stick to a schedule when teaching these tasks; progress will take time and should not be rushed.

The section on management of low back pain, as opposed to treatment, is especially valuable. A well thought-out prospective clinical reasoning process will occasionally lead to the conclusion that physical treatment may not be effective. To recognize this is not to admit defeat. On the contrary, our understanding of the underlying pathology puts us in an ideal position to educate and to refer appropriately. As one of my former professors noted with great annoyance, "If physiotherapy is not indicated, then it is by definition contraindicated!". Our profession's standing in the medical community will be improved if we intervene only in cases where we will be effective.

There is a need for standardized, clinically applicable classification systems for lumbar dysfunction for numerous reasons: as a method of diagnosing the problem, to establish a prognosis, to provide a base for quality outcome research, and not least of all to enable us as physiotherapists to communicate with each other without jargon getting in the way. Designing such a system is a difficult task and the authors are to be commended on their proposal. It will be interesting to see if their system holds up to use clinically as well as in the realm of research.

My criticisms with the clinical application of the SDM are few, and have to do with the application of manual therapy. The authors certainly advocate a well-applied manual assessment to determine the level of dysfunction, and use a manual approach to deal with a lack of movement at adjoining segments. This is certainly not an 'exercise-only' model of treatment, nor should it be. The stated goal of treatment is not primarily pain control, but control of abnormal movement; therefore, mobilization of the affected segment is contraindicated by the authors for numerous reasons. I believe that pain control and motor retraining are inextricably linked.

The application of manual therapy has traditionally been based on spinal biomechanics; however, recent research shows improvements following manual treatment owe more to complex connections in the central nervous system than to joint biomechanics (1). If we consider dysfunction in the segmental control musculature a reaction to pain at the affected segment (2), and judiciously applied manual therapy reduces pain (1), cannot motor learning and muscle activation be enhanced by pain reduction?

Overall, this is an excellent clinical model. The view that the majority of people with low back pain require motor retraining is not overly-dogmatic; it is based more and more in scientific fact. The authors' paradigm should be embraced by practicing clinicians.

References

1. Malisza KL, Gregorash L, Turner A, Foniok T, Stroman P, Allman A, Summers R and Wright A (2003) Functional MRI involving painful stimulation of the ankle and the effect of physiotherapy joint mobilization. Magnetic Resonance Imaging. 21(5), 489-496

2. Hides J, Stokes M, Saide M, *et al*. Evidence of lumbar multifidus muscle wasting ipsilateral to symptoms in patients with acute/subacute low back pain. *Spine* 1994;19:165–72

glossary

Active Subsystem

Panjabi developed the term 'active subsystem' to describe the various trunk muscles which generate the segmental stiffness necessary to control segmental motion and maintain normal neutral zone amplitudes. The muscles of the active subsystem dissipate spinal loads such that osseoligamentous and neural tissues do not become injured.

Adaptive Model of Altered Motor Control in Lumbar Pathology

The motor control changes which develop in the setting of lumbar pathology may be interpreted as being adaptive or beneficial. The adaptive model recognizes that a wide variety of trunk muscles have the potential to generate spinal stiffness such that the Euler stability (see definition below) of the lumbar spine is maintained. This interpretation emphasizes the beneficial aspects of the motor control changes which occur in the superficial or multi-segmental muscles in the presence of lumbar pathology.

Arthrokinematics

The theoretical motions which occur between joint surfaces during physiological movement. In the lumbar spine arthrokinematic movements occur at the interbody and zygapophysial joints.

Biomechanical Models

A biomechanical model is a mathematical representation of a biological system. In the context of the lumbar spine, a variety of functions or behaviours of the normal and pathological spine may be modeled using mathematical equations. Biomechanical models may be static or dynamic with static models being less biologically robust.

Biopsychosocial Model of Lumbar Pathology

This model considers the interactions of biological, psychological, cognitive, behavioural and sociocultural factors and their impact on pain and disability in the setting of lumbar pathology.

Catastrophization

A systematic distortion of information from the environment. This schema leads the individual to anticipate the worst possible outcome for an event or to misinterpret an event as an utter catastrophe. A patient who catastrophizes about low back pain would tend to interpret this noxious stimulus as terrible, overwhelming, and tragic (Burns et al., 1999).

Central Sensitization

The sensitization of pain-modulating systems in the central nervous system at both spinal and supraspinal levels. Central sensitization is facilitated by numerous parameters that contribute to the maintenance of pain and which vary from individual to individual. Briefly, the 'sensitized' central nervous system evolves to a state where pain is more easily and frequently experienced by the individual.

Chiropractic

A system of complementary medicine based on the diagnosis and manipulative treatment of misalignments of the joints, especially those of the spinal column, which are held to cause other disorders by affecting the nerves, muscles, and organs (Pearsall et al, 1998).

Clinical Instability

Any circumstance which results in a significant decrease in the ability of the spinal stabilization system to maintain the intervertebral neutral zone(s) within physiological limits such that there is no neurological dysfunction, no major deformity and no incapacitating pain (Panjabi, 1992).

Clinical Reasoning

The processes by which the clinician, through interaction with the patient and other significant stakeholders, structures meaning, goals and health management strategies based on clinical data, client choices as well as professional judgment and knowledge (Higgs & Jones, 2000). Broadly, clinical reasoning refers to the multi-dimensional cognitive processes by which clinicians develop accurate diagnoses and best-practice plans of patient management.

Connective Tissue Compliance (Segmental Compliance)

As utilized throughout this text, segmental or connective tissue compliance refers to the degree of 'give' or the ease with which a motion segment distends secondary to a manually applied pressure. In this context, segmental compliance may also be considered as the reciprocal of segmental stiffness.

Cross Talk

A casual term describing the problem of signal contamination in surface electromyography (SEMG) applications. Specifically, it refers to the tendency for SEMG to record from muscles other than the target muscle in addition to the target muscle. Cross talk is a function of volume conduction and the SEMG receptive field.

Differential Activation

A term referring to the temporal differences in recruitment observed within a group of muscles or within a single muscle during functional movements. In a rehabilitation context, the restoration of normal or near-normal differential activation is approached by instructing the patient in specific patterns of voluntary activation or contraction of selected trunk muscles using a variety of feedback tools.

Differential Diagnosis

Frequently, a patient's signs and symptoms are consistent with two or more pathological conditions. The term 'differential' diagnosis refers to the process by which the clinician arrives at a definitive diagnosis under such circumstances. This requires the clinician to utilize a strategy in which both the subjective and objective examinations are structured to elicit sufficient evidence to confirm a single diagnostic hypothesis and negate other potential diagnoses.

Direct Manipulation Technique

The term 'direct' technique applies to any mobilization or manipulation technique whereby the manual force is applied to the side of the spine ipsilateral or closest to the clinician. For example, if the patient is in right side-lying, a direct technique would deliver the force to the left side of the target motion segment. Direct techniques are considered appropriate when there are no other segments in the region which are symptomatic in the same direction as that being restored via the mobilization or manipulation.

Discogenic low back pain

A casual term, rooted in the pathoanatomical model, used to describe the situation where a patient's symptoms are believed to be secondary to some form of pathology affecting the intervertebral disc.

Elastic Zone

"That part of the physiological intervertebral motion, measured from the end of the neutral zone up to the physiological limit. Within the EZ spinal motion is produced against a significant internal resistance" (Panjabi, 1992).

Euler Stability

Euler, a Swiss mathematician (1707 - 1783), developed a set of equations to predict the stability of vertical structures or columns. These equations are still in wide use today within the engineering profession. Euler stability is concerned with the ability of a column to withstand load and avoid collapse or buckling. In this context, the stability of the structure is proportionate to its stiffness, the greater the stiffness, the greater the stability.

Form and Force Closure Model

Andre Vleeming and colleagues at Erasmus University in Rotterdam developed the form and force closure model which describes the stabilizing mechanisms acting at the joints of the pelvis. Under this model, form closure refers to the stability afforded the pelvis via the structure of its joints while force closure refers to the stability provided by the musculofascial systems acting at the pelvis.

Hypervigilance

A behavioural state in which the individual pays an inordinate amount of attention to somatic sensations, ever attentive to the potential onset of pain.

Hypothetico-deductive process

Considered a mainstay of the scientific method, the hypothetico-deductive model refers to the systematic process by which a clinical diagnosis is initially formed, then challenged, tested and eventually either confirmed or refuted via the subjective and objective examinations.

Indirect Manipulation Technique

The term 'indirect' technique applies to any mobilization or manipulation technique whereby the manual force is applied to the side of the spine contralateral to the clinician. For example, if the patient is in right side-lying, an indirect technique would deliver the force to the right side of the target motion segment. Indirect techniques are considered appropriate when other segments in the region are symptomatic in the same direction as that being restored *via* the mobilization or manipulation.

Inner Unit

A term developed to define a set of muscles considered by some to be critical to lumbopelvic stability – the transversus abdominis, multifidus, pelvic floor and diaphragm (Lee, 1999).

Maladaptive Model of Altered Motor Control in Lumbar Pathology

The motor control changes which develop in the setting of lumbar pathology may be interpreted as being maladaptive or deleterious. The maladaptive model emphasizes the proposed negative effects of the motor control changes in both the segmental and multi-segmental muscles. The neuro-physiological alterations in muscles such as transversus abdominis, deep multifidus and the superficial multi-segmental muscles are seen as being detrimental in terms of segmental motion control, spinal loading and respiratory function.

Motion Segment

Also known as a mobile segment or a functional spinal unit, the term motion segment refers to any two adjacent vertebrae, their shared intervertebral disc and the ligaments which act at that segment. The passive elements of any muscles which act at the segment may also be considered a component of the motion segment.

Neurodynamics

The mechanical properties of neural tissues pertaining to the ability of these tissues to tolerate loading as associated with physiological movements of the axial and peripheral skeleton.

Neutral Position

As defined by Panjabi, the neutral position (NP) is 'the posture of the spine in which the overall internal stresses in the spinal column and the muscular effort to hold the posture are minimal'. Experimentally, the NP is defined as the point in range half-way between the two opposing boundaries of the neutral zone (NZ) at opposite ends of the same plane of movement (eg., the 'extension' NZ and the 'flexion' NZ in the sagittal plane). It is important for clinicians to appreciate that this *in vitro* NP is not analogous to the *in vivo* neutral position of the lumbar spine.

Neutral Zone

The neutral zone (NZ) is that component of the *in vitro* physiological ROM through which spinal segmental motion occurs against minimal internal or osseoligamentous resistance; as such, it is a zone of minimal stiffness or high laxity (Panjabi, 1992). Movement through the *in vivo* NZ is expected to encounter markedly greater stiffness secondary to the stabilizing effect of muscle generated *via* increased intersegmental compression.

Organic Pathology

This somewhat casual term is used to denote pathology with an identifiable, physical etiology. Conversely, the term 'non-organic' is used to define conditions or symptoms believed to be psychogenic in origin.

Pathoanatomical Model

A traditional conceptualization of pathology in which one or more anatomical structure(s) is presumed to be the source of the patient's symptoms. In the context of lumbar pathology, pathoanatomical diagnoses include facet joint syndrome, lumbar strain, disc herniation and degenerative disc disease.

Pilates

An approach to exercise developed throughout the 1920's by Joseph Pilates. Pilates, in combining his interests in yoga, Zen meditation and martial arts with his background in gymnastics, diving and boxing, devised a unique sequence of movements which he felt improved both muscular endurance and flexibility. His approach was originally popular within the professional dance community and has recently become a widespread fitness phenomena.

Prospective Clinical Reasoning

An approach to diagnosis based on pattern recognition and the hypothetico-deductive process. Upon initial contact with the patient, the clinician begins formulating potential diagnoses and engages in a process of real-time hypothesis formulation and testing. A patient-specific subjective examination is used to develop a differential diagnosis while the objective or physical examination is utilized to confirm the differential diagnosis.

Proximate and Ultimate Factors

In terms of cause and effect relationships, a proximate factor is one which is most immediately related to the onset of an event. Ultimate factors are those which lead to or result in these proximate factors. In his book 'Guns, Germs and Steel' Jared Diamond discusses the forces which shaped the evolution and extinction of early human societies. In one example, the decimation of thousands of crudely equipped South American warriors by a few hundred Spanish on horseback wielding metal swords provides the context for an examination of proximate and ultimate factors. The proximate factors around this situation included the superior weapons of the Spaniards. The ultimate factors involved the social and environmental realities which led to the fact that the Spanish had such weapons while the South Americans did not.

Receptive Field

A term used to define the volume of tissue from which a surface electromyography device may capture bioelectric signals. The size of this field is a function of the size of the recording electrode, the distance between the recording electrodes, the orientation of the recording electrodes relative to the muscle's fibre direction, the phenomena of volume conduction and the degree of muscle activation or recruitment. The receptive field is not limited to the first layer of muscle tissue directly under the recording electrodes.

Retrospective Clinical Reasoning

An approach to diagnosis whereby both the subjective and physical examinations are utilized to gather data. The clinician typically asks a great number of questions and performs as many region-specific tests as they can in order to generate the greatest amount of patient information. Theoretically, there is no attempt to form a diagnosis until both components of the examination are completed.

Segmental Integrity Test

A manual therapy technique utilized to develop an appreciation for the stiffness or compliance of the spine when a uni-planar force or load is applied to the spine at a specific motion segment. Traditionally, these tests have been termed 'stability' tests; however, given the multi-system nature of spinal stability, the authors feel it inappropriate to refer to such techniques as 'stability' tests.

Volume Conduction

As a muscle contracts, biologically generated voltage differentials spread throughout the conductive membranes of the active muscle as well as through adjacent conductive tissues. This 'volume conduction', along with the relatively large size of the receptive field of the surface electromyogram, is responsible for the fact that signals captured by surface electromyography cannot be solely attributed to any single muscle. Typically, the SEMG signal is a composite of electrical activity arising from a variety of potential sources, including, but not limited to, the target muscle.

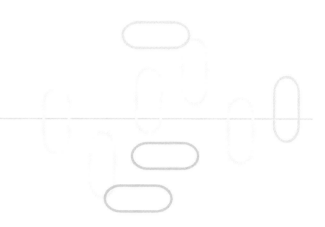

references

Andersson EA, Oddsson L, Nilsson J, Grundstrom H, Thorstensson A. EMG activities of the quadratus lumborum and erector spinae muscles during flexion-relaxation and other motor tasks. Clin Biomech 1996 Oct 11(7):392 – 400

Aruin AS, Latash ML. Directional specificity of postural muscles in feed-forward postural reactions during fast voluntary arm movements. Exp Brain Res 1995 103:323 – 332

Barker KL, Shamley DR, Jackson D. Changes in the cross-sectional area of multifidus and psoas in patients with unilateral back pain. Spine 2004 29 (22): E515 – E519

Barker PJ, Briggs CA. Attachments of the posterior layer of lumbar fascia. Spine 1999 24 (17):1757 – 1764

Barker PJ, Briggs CA, Bogeski G. Tensile transmission across the lumbar fasciae in unembalmed cadavers. Spine 2004 29 (2):129 – 138

Bergmark A. Stability of the lumbar spine. A study in mechanical engineering. Acta Orthop Scand Suppl. 1989 230:1 - 54

Bergquist-Ullman M, Larsson U. Acute low back pain in industry. A controlled prospective study with special reference to therapy and confounding factors. Acta Orthop Scand 1977 (170):1-117

Bogduk N, Macintosh JE. The applied anatomy of the thoracolumbar fascia. Spine 1984 9 (2):164 – 170

Bogduk N(a). Clinical anatomy of the lumbar spine and sacrum, 3rd Ed. 1997 Churchill Livngstone, Edinburgh p. 14

Bogduk N(b). Clinical anatomy of the lumbar spine and sacrum, 3rd Ed. 1997 Churchill Livngstone, Edinburgh pp. 95— 97

Bogduk N(c). Clinical anatomy of the lumbar spine and sacrum, 3rd Ed. 1997 Churchill Livngstone, Edinburgh p. 96

Bogduk N, Mercer S. Biomechanics of the cervical spine. I: Normal kinematics. Clin Biomech 2000 15:633 – 648

Bogduk N. Management of chronic low back pain. MJA 2004 180 (19):79— 83

Borkan J, Koes B, Reis S, et al. A report from the second international forum for primary care research on low back pain: reexamining priorities. Spine 1998 23 (18):1992 – 1996

Bouter L, Pennick V, Bombardier C. Cochrane back review group. Spine 2003 28 (12):1215 – 1218

Bronfort G, Haas M, Evans RL, Bouter L. Efficacy of spinal manipulation and mobilization for low back pain and neck pain: a systematic review and best evidence synthesis. Spine J. 2004 4 (3):335 - 356

Brox JI, Sorensen R, Friis A, Nygaard O, Indahl A, Keller A, Ingebrigsten T, Eriksen HR, Holm I, Koller AK, Riise R, Reikeras O. Randomized clinical trial of lumbar instrumented fusion and cognitive intervention and exercises in patients with chronic low back pain and disc degeneration. Spine 2003 28 (17):1913 – 1921

Butler DS. The sensitive nervous system. 2000 Noigroup Publications, Adelaide Australia

Butler DS, Moseley GL. Explain pain. 2003 Noigroup Publications, Adelaide Australia

Carr JH, Shepherd RB. Physiotherapy in disorders of the brain. 1980 William Heinemann Medical Books Limited, London, UK p. 73

Charlin B, Tardif J, Boshuizen HPA. Scripts and medical diagnostic knowledge: Theory and applications for clinical reasoning instruction and research. Acad Med 2000 75 (2): 182 – 190

Cholewicki J, McGill S, Norman RW. Lumbar spine load during the lifting of extremely heavy weights. Med Sci Sports Exerc 1991 23 (10):1179 - 1186

Cholewicki J, McGill SM. Lumbar posterior ligament involvement during extremely heavy lifts estimated from fluoroscopic measurements. J Biomech 1992 25 (1):17 – 28

Cholewicki J, McGill SM. Mechanical stability of the *in vivo* lumbar spine: implications for injury and chronic low back pain. Clin Biomech 1996 11 (1):1 – 15

Cholewicki J, Crisco JJ, Oxland TR, Yamamoto I, Panjabi MM. Effects of posture and structure on three-dimensional coupled rotations in the lumbar spine. Spine 1996 21 (21): 2421 - 2428

Cholewicki J, Panjabi MM, Khachatryan A. Stabilizing function of trunk flexor-extensor muscles around a neutral spine posture. Spine 1997 22 (19):2207 – 2212

Cholewicki J, van Dieen JH, Arsenault AB. Muscle function and dysfunction in the spine. J EMG Kines 2003 (13):303 – 304

Comerford MJ, Mottram SL. Movement and stability dysfunction - contemporary developments. Man Ther 2001 6 (1):15 - 26

Cook C. Coupling behaviour of the lumbar spine: A literature review. J Man Manip Ther 2003 11 (3):137 – 145

Cook C, Showalter C. A survey on the importance of lumbar coupling biomechanics in physiotherapy practice. Man Ther 2004 Aug (3):162 - 172

Coppieters MW, Kurz K, Mortensen TE, Richards NL, Skaret IA, McLaughlin LM, Hodges PW. The impact of neurodynamic testing on the perception of experimentally induced muscle pain. Man Ther 2005 10 (1): 52-60.

Cresswell AG, Oddsson L, Thorstensson A. The influence of sudden perturbations on trunk muscle activity and intra-abdominal pressure while standing. Exp Brain Res 1994 (98):336 – 341

Crisco JJ. The biomechanical stability of the human lumbar spine: experimental and theoretical investigations. 1989 Doctoral dissertation, Yale University, New Haven CT

Crisco JJ, Panjabi, MM. The intersegmental and multisegmental muscles of the lumbar spine. A biomechanical model comparing lateral stabilizing potential. Spine 1991 16 (7):793 – 799

Crisco JJ, Panjabi MM, Yamamoto I, Oxland TR. Euler stability of the human ligamentous lumbar spine. Clin Biomech 1992 7 (1):27— 32

Critchley D. Instructing pelvic floor contraction facilitates transversus abdominis thickness increase during low-abdominal hollowing. Physiother Res Int. 2002 7 (2): 65 - 75

Croft PR, Macfarlane GJ, Papageorgiou AC, Thomas E, Silman AJ. Outcome of low back pain in general practice: a prospective study. Br Med J 1998 (316): 1356 – 1359

Custers EJFM, Stuyt PMJ, De Vries Robbe PF. Clinical Problem Analysis (CPA): A systematic approach to teaching complex medical problem solving. Acad Med 2000 75 (3): 291 – 297

Cyriax, J. Textbook of Orthopaedic Medicine, Volume 1. Diagnosis of Soft Tissue Lesions. Eastbourne, UK. Bailliere Tindall, 1982 pp 53 – 54.

Daemen MA, Kurvers HA, Kitslaar PJ, Slaaf DW, Bullens PH, Van den Wildenberg FA. Neurogenic inflammation in an animal model of neuropathic pain. Neurol Res. 1998 20 (1):41 - 45

Dangaria TR, Naesh O. Changes in cross-sectional area of psoas major muscle in unilateral sciatica caused by disc herniation. Spine 1998 23 (8):928 – 931

Danneels LA, Vanderstraeten GG, Cambier DC, Witvrouw EE, De Cuyper HJ. CT imaging of trunk muscles in chronic low back pain patients and healthy control subjects. Eur Spine J 2000 (9):266 – 272

Danneels LA, Cagnie BJ, Cools AM, Vanderstraeten GG, Cambier DC, Witvrouw EE, De Cuyper HJ. Intra-operator and inter-operator reliability of surface electromyography in the clinical evaluation of back muscles. Man Ther 2001 6 (3):145 – 153

deAndrade JR, Grant C, Dixon AS. Joint distension and reflex muscle inhibition in the knee. J Bone Joint Surg Am 1965 (47):313 - 322

Delp SL, Suryanarayanan S, Murray WM, Uhlir J, Triolo RJ. Architecture of the rectus abdominis, quadratus lumborum and erector spinae. J Biomech 2001 (34):371 – 375

Devor M, Seltzer Z. Pathophysiology of damaged nerves in relation to chronic pain. *In*: Textbook of Pain. 4th Ed. Wall PD, Melzack R (eds) (1999) Churchill Livingstone

Doubell TP, Mannion R, Woolf CJ. The dorsal horn: state dependent sensory processing, plasticity and the generation of pain. In: Textbook of Pain. 4th Ed. Wall PD, Melzack R (eds) (1999) Churchill Livingstone)

Drinkwater M. personal communication, 2003

Elstein AS, Shulman LS, Sprafka SA. Medical problem solving: An analysis of clinical reasoning. 1978 Harvard University Press, Cambridge, MA

Ferreira PH, Ferreira ML, Hodges PW. Changes in recruitment of the abdominal muscles in people with low back pain. Spine 2004 29 (22):2560 - 2566

Fransen M, Woodward M, Norton R, Coggan C, Dawe M, Sheridan N. Risk factors associated with the transition from acute to chronic occupational back pain. Spine. 2002 27(1):92-98

Fritz, J. Use of a classification approach to the treatment of 3 patients with low back syndrome. Phys Ther 1998 78 (7): 766 - 782

Frost H, Lamb SE, Doll HA, Taffe-Carver P, Stewart-Brown S. Randomised controlled trial of physiotherapy compared with advice for low back pain. BMJ 2004 (329): 708 - 714

Fryette H. The principles of osteopathic technique. Academy of Applied Osteopathy; Carmel CA 1954 pp. 1 – 14

Ferguson SA, Marras WS, Burr DL, Davis KG, Gupta P. Differences in motor recruitment and resulting kinematics between low back pain patients and asymptomatic participants during lifting exertions. Clin Biomech 2004 (19):992 - 999

Gertzbein SD, Seligman J, Holtby R, Chan KH, Kapasouri A, Tile M, Cruickshank B. Centrode patterns and segmental instability in degenerative disc disease. Spine 1985 10 (3): 257 – 261

Gertzbein SD, Seligman J, Holtby R, Chan KW, Ogston

N, Kapasouri A, Tile M. Centrode characteristics of the lumbar spine as a function of segmental instability. Clin Ortho Rel Res 1986 (208):48 – 51

Gibbons S. Biomechanics and stability mechanisms of psoas major. *In*, Proceedings of the 4th Interdisciplinary World Congress on Low Back & Pelvic Pain. Montreal, 2001 pp. 246 – 247

Haggmark T, Thorstensson A. Fibre types in human abdominal muscles. Acta Physiol Scand 1979 107 (4):319 - 325

Herzog W, Ed. Clinical biomechanics of spinal manipulation. 2000 Churchill Livingstone, Edinburgh, UK

Hickling J, Maitland GD. Abnormalities in passive movement: diagrammatic representation. Physiotherapy. 1970 56 (3):105 - 114

Hides JA, Stokes MJ, Saide M, Jull GA, Cooper DH. Evidence of lumbar multifidus muscle wasting ipsilateral to symptoms in patients with acute/subacute low back pain. Spine 1994 19 (2):165 – 172

Hides JA, Richardson CA, Jull GA. Multifidus muscle recovery is not automatic after resolution of acute, first-episode low back pain. Spine 1996 21 (23):2763 – 2769

Hides JA, Jull GA, Richardson CA. Long-term effects of specific stabilizing exercises for first-episode low back pain. Spine 2001 26 (11): E243 – E248

Hodges PW, Richardson CA. Inefficient muscular stabilization of the lumbar spine associated with low back pain. A motor control evaluation of transversus abdominis. Spine 1996 21 (22):2640 – 2649

Hodges PW, Richardson CA(a).Contraction of the abdominal muscles associated with movement of the lower limb. Phys Ther 1997 77 (2):132 - 143

Hodges PW, Richardson CA(b). Feedforward contraction of transversus abdominis is not influenced by the direction of arm movement. Exp Brain Res 1997 (114):362 – 370

Hodges PW, Richardson CA. Delayed postural contraction of transversus abdominis in low back pain associated with movement of the lower limb. J Spinal Disord. 1998 11(1): 46 - 56

Hodges PW, Cresswell A, Thorstensson A. Preparatory trunk motion accompanies rapid upper limb movement. Exp Brain Res 1999 (124):69 – 79

Hodges PW. Changes in motor planning of feedforward postural responses of the trunk muscles in low back pain. Exp Brain Res 2001 (141):261 – 266

Hodges PW. Core stability exercises in chronic low back pain. Ortho Clin N Am 2003 34 (2):245 - 254

Hodges PW, Moseley GL. Pain and motor control of the lumbopelvic region: effect and possible mechanisms. J EMG Kines 2003 (13):361 – 370

Hodges PW, Kaigle-Holm A, Holm S, Ekstrom L, Cresswell A, Hansson T, Thorstensson A. Intervertebral stiffness of the spine is increased by evoked contraction of transversus abdominis and the diaphragm: In vivo porcine studies. Spine 2003 28 (23):2594 – 2601

Hodges PW. Interventions aimed at improving the control and coordination of the spine. *In*, Proceedings of the 5th Interdisciplinary World Congress on Low Back & Pelvic Pain. Melbourne, 2004

Holtby R, Razmjou H. Accuracy of the Speed's and Yergason's tests in detecting biceps pathology and SLAP lesions: comparison with arthroscopic findings. Arthroscopy 2004 20(3):231 - 236

Hoogendoorn WE, van Poppel MNM, Bongers PM, Koes BW, Bouter LM. Systematic review of psychosocial factors at work and private life as risk factors for back pain. Spine 2000 25 (16):2114 – 2125

Hurley DA, McDonough SM, Dempster M, Moore AP, Baxter GD. A randomized clinical trial of manipulative therapy and interferential therapy for acute low back pain. Spine 2004 29 (20):2207 - 2216

Indahl A, Kaigle AM, Reikeras O, Holm SH. Interaction between the porcine lumbar intervertebral disc, zygapophysial joints, and paraspinal muscles. Spine 1997 22 (24):2834 – 2840

Jemmett RS. Rehabilitation of lumbar multifidus dysfunction in low back pain: strengthening versus a motor re-education model. 2003 Br J Sports Med 37 (1):91 - 92

Jemmett RS, MacDonald DA, Agur AMR. Anatomical relationships between selected segmental muscles of the lumbar spine in the context of multi-planar segmental motion: A preliminary investigation. Man Ther 2004 9 (4): 203-10

Jones MA. Clinical reasoning in manual therapy. Phys Ther 1992 72 (12):875 – 884

Jones MA. Clinical reasoning: the foundation of clinical practice. Part 1. Aus Physiother 1997 43 (3):167 – 169

Kader DF, Wardlaw D, Smith FW. Correlation between the MRI changes in the lumbar multifidus muscles and leg pain. Clin Radiol 2000 (55):145 – 149

Kaigle AM, Holm SH, Hansson TH. Experimental instability in the lumbar spine. Spine 1995 20 (4):421 – 430

Kasman G. Course Notes: Surface EMG & Biofeedback in Physical Therapy. 1996

Keller A, Gunderson R, Reikeras O, Brox JI. Reliability of computed tomography measurements of paraspinal muscle cross-sectional area and density in patiernts with chronic low back pain. Spine 2003 28 (13):1455 – 1460

Knuttson F. The instability associated with disk degeneration in the lumbar spine. Acta Radio 1944 (25): 593 – 608

Koes, B. Acute low back pain: Presentation of the new European guidelines. *In*, Proceedings of the 5th Interdisciplinary World Congress on Low Back & Pelvic Pain. Melbourne, 2004

Krause N, Ragland DR, Fisher JM, Syme SL. Psychosocial job factors, physical workload and incidence of work-related spinal injury: A 5 year prospective study of urban transit operators. Spine 1998 23 (23):2507 – 2516

Kulig K, Landel R, Powers CM. Assessment of lumbar spine kinematics using dynamic MRI: a proposed mechanism of sagittal motion induced by manual posterior to anterior mobilization. J Ortho Sports Ther 2004 (34):57 – 64

Laslett, M. Validity of the clinical examination in chronic

low back pain. *In*, Proceedings of the 5th Interdisciplinary World Congress on Low Back & Pelvic Pain. Melbourne, 2004

Lee D(a). The pelvic girdle: An approach to the examination and treatment of the lumbo-pelvic-hip region 2nd Ed. 1999 Churchill Livingstone, London pp. 28 – 29

Lee D(b). The pelvic girdle: An approach to the examination and treatment of the lumbo-pelvic-hip region 2nd Ed. 1999 Churchill Livingstone, London pp. 58 - 60

Lee D(c). The pelvic girdle: An approach to the examination and treatment of the lumbo-pelvic-hip region 2nd Ed. 1999 Churchill Livingstone, London pp. 160 - 162

Lee D(d). The pelvic girdle: An approach to the examination and treatment of the lumbo-pelvic-hip region 2nd Ed. 1999 Churchill Livingstone, London pp. 96 - 97

Lee RYW, Evans JH. An in vivo study of the intervertebral movements produced by posterioranterior mobilisation. Clin Biomech 1997 (12):400 – 408

Lee RYW, McGregor AH, Bull AMJ, Wragg P. Dynamic response of the cervical spine to posterioranterior mobilization. Clin Biomech 2005 20 (2): 228 - 231

Lucas DB, Bresler B. Stability of the ligamentous spine. 1961 Biomechanics Laboratory, University of Southern California, # 40

MacDonald DA, Hodges PW, Moseley L. The function of the lumbar multifidus in unilateral low back pain. *In*, Proceedings of the 5th Interdisciplinary World Congress on Low Back & Pelvic Pain. Melbourne, 2004

Macintosh JE, Valencia F, Bogduk N, Munro RR. The morphology of the lumbar multifidus muscles. Clin Biomech 1986 1:196 – 204

MacIntosh JE, Bogduk N. The biomechanics of the lumbar multifidus. Clin Biomech 1986 1 :205 – 213

Macintosh JE, Bogduk N. The morphology of the lumbar erector spinae. Spine 1987 12 (7):658 - 668

Macintosh JE, Bogduk N. The attachments of the lumbar erector spinae. Spine. 1991 16 (7):783 - 792

MacNab I. Negative disc exploration; an analysis of the causes of nerve-root involvement in sixty eight patients. J Bone Joint Surg 53A 1971 (5):891 – 903

MacNab I. In, *Backache* 1977 Williams & Wilkins, Baltimore; p 4- 7

Mannion, AF. Prevention of low back pain: Presentation of the new European guidelines. *In*, Proceedings of the 5th Interdisciplinary World Congress on Low Back & Pelvic Pain. Melbourne, 2004

Mannion AF, Muntener M, Taimela S, Dvorak J. A randomized clinical trial of three active therapies for chronic low back pain. Spine 1999 24 (23):2435 – 2448

Marras WS, Davis KG, Ferguson SA, Lucas BR, Gupta P. Spine loading characteristics of patients with low back pain compared with asymptomatic individuals. Spine 2001 26 (23):2566 – 2574

McGill SM, Norman RW. Partitioning of the L4-L5 dynamic moment into disc, ligamentous and muscular components during lifting. Spine 1986 11 (7):666 – 677

McGill SM, Juker D, Kropf P. Quantitative intramuscular myoelectric activity of quadratus lumborum during a wide variety of tasks. Clin Biomech 1996 11 (3):170 – 172

McGill SM. The biomechanics of low back injury: Implications on current practice in industry and the clinic. J Biomech 1997 30 (5):465 – 475

McGill SM(a). Low back disorders. Evidence-based prevention and rehabilitation. 2002 Human Kinetics Champaign, Ill. p. 138

McGill SM(b). Low back disorders. Evidence-based prevention and rehabilitation. 2002 Human Kinetics Champaign, Ill. ch. 13

McGill SM(c). Low back disorders. Evidence-based prevention and rehabilitation. 2002 Human Kinetics Champaign, Ill. pp. 12 - 15

McGill SM, Grenier S, Kavcic N, Cholewicki J. Coordination of muscle activity to assure stability of the lumbar spine. J EMG Kines 2003 (13):353 – 359

McGlashen K, Miller J, Schultz A, Andersson G. Load-displacement behavior of the human lumbo-sacral joint. J Ortho Res 1987 (5):488 – 498

McMeeken JM, Beith ID, Newham DJ, Milligan P, Critchley DJ. The relationship between EMG and change in thickness of transversus abdominis. Clin Biomech 2004 19 (4):337 - 342

Meadows J. personal communication, 2001

Mimura M, Moriya H, Watanabe T, Takahashi K, Yamagata M, Tamaki T. Three-dimensional motion analysis of the cervical spine with special reference to the axial rotation. Spine 1989 14 (11):1135 – 1139

Moller H, Sundin A, Hedlund R. Symptoms, signs and functional disability in adult spondylolisthesis. Spine 2000 25 (6):683 – 689

Mooney V. The classification of low back pain. Ann Med. 1989 21 (5):321 - 325

Moseley L, Hodges PW, Gandevia SC. Deep and superficial fibers of the lumbar multifidus are differentially active during voluntary arm movements. Spine 2002 27 (2):E29 – E36

Moseley L, Hodges PW, Gandevia SC. External perturbation of the trunk in standing humans differentially activates components of the medial back muscles. J Physiol 2003 547(Part 2):581-587

Moseley, L. Combined physiotherapy and education is efficacious for chronic low back pain. Aust J Physiother 2002 48 (4):297-302

Moseley L. A pain neuromatrix approach to patients with chronic pain. Man Ther 2003 8 (3):130-40

Murphy PL, Courtney TK. Low back pain disability: relative costs by antecedent and industry group. Am J Ind Med. 2000 37(5):558-571

Nachemson AL. Advances in low-back pain. Clin Orthop. 1985 (200):266 - 278

Neumann P, Gill V. Pelvic floor and abdominal muscleinteraction: EMG activity and intra-abdominal pressure. Int Urogynecol J Pelvic Floor Dysfunct. 2002 13 (2):125 – 132

Niemisto L, Lahtinen-Suopanki T, Rissanen P, Lindgren KA, Sarna S, Hurri H. A randomized trial of combined manipulation, stabilizing exercises and physician consultation compared to physician consultation alone for chronic low back pain. Spine 2003 28 (19):2185 – 2191

Olson MW, Li L, Solomonow M. Flexion-relaxation response to cyclic lumbar flexion. Clin Biomech 2004 (19):769 - 776

O'Sullivan PB, Twomey LT, Allison GT. Evaluation of specific stabilizing exercise in the treatment of chronic low back pain with radiologic diagnosis of spondylolysis or spondylolisthesis. Spine 1997 22 (24):2959 - 2967

O'Sullivan PB. Lumbar segmental 'instability': clinical presentation and specific stabilizing exercise management. Man Ther 2000 5 (1):2 – 12

Oxland TR, Panjabi MM. The onset and progression of spinal injury: a demonstration of neutral zone sensitivity. J Biomech 1992 25 (10):1165 – 1172

Panjabi, MM. Experimental determination of spinal motion segment behaviour. Ortho Clin N Am 1977 8 (1):169 – 180

Panjabi MM, Abumi K, Duranceau J, Oxland TR. Spinal stability and intersegmental muscle forces. A biomechanical model. Spine 1989 14 (2):194 – 200

Panjabi MM, Yamamoto I, Oxland TR, Crisco JJ. How does posture affect coupling in the lumbar spine. Spine 1989 14 (9):1002 - 1111

Panjabi MM(a). The stabilizing system of the spine. Part I. Function, dysfunction , adaptation and enhancement. J Spinal Disorders 1992 5 (4):383 – 389

Panjabi MM(b). The stabilizing system of the spine. Part II. Neutral zone and instability hypothesis. J Spinal Disorders 1992 5 (4):390 – 397

Panjabi MM, Oxland TR, Yamamoto I Crisco JJ. Mechanical behavior of the human lumbar and lumbosacral spine as shown by three-dimensional load-displacement curves. Am J Bone & Joint Surg 1994 (76):413 - 424

Panjabi MM, Kifune M, Liou W, Arand M, Vasavada A, Oxland TR. Graded thoracolumbar spinal injuries: development of multidirectional instability. Eur Spine J 1998 (7):332 – 339

Panjabi MM. Clinical spinal instability and low back pain. J EMG Kines 2003 (13):371 – 379

Parkkola R, Rytokoski U, Kormano M. Magnetic resonance imaging of the discs and trunk muscles in patients with chronic low back pain and healthy control subjects. Spine 1993 18 (7):830-836

Pearcy M, Tibrewal M. Axial rotation and lateral bending in the normal lumbar spine measured by three dimensional radiography. Spine 1984 9 (6):582 – 587

Pearsall J. The New Oxford Dictionary of English. Oxford University Press, London, 1998

Pettman E. V4 Course Notes. 2000 Canadian Physiotherapy Association; Orthopaedic Division. Ottawa, ON

Pincus T, Burton AK, Vogel S, Field AP. A systematic review of psychosocial factors as predictors of chronicity/disability in prospective cohorts of low back pain. Spine 2002 27 (5): E109-E120

Pincus T, Vlaeyen JWS, Kendall NAS, Von Korff MR, Kalauokalani DA, Reis S. Cognitive-behavioral therapy and psychosocial factors in low back pain. Spine 2002 27 (5): E133 – E138

Pool-Goudzwaard AL, Vleeming A, Stoeckart R, Snijders CJ, Mens JMA. Insufficient lumbopelvic stability: a clinical,anatomical and biomechanical approach to 'a-specific' low back pain. Man Ther 1998 3 (10):12 – 20

Powers CM, Kulig K, Harrison J, Bergman G. Segmental mobility of the lumbar spine during a posterior to anterior mobilization: assessment using dynamic MRI. Clin Biomech 2003 (18):80 - 83

Preuss R, Fung J. Can acute low back pain result from segmental spinal buckling during sub-maximal activities? A review of the current literature. Man Ther 2005 10 (1): 14-20

Quint U, Wilke HJ, Shirazi-Adl A, Parnianpour M, Loer F, Claes LE. Importance of the intersegmental trunk muscles for the stability of the lumbar spine. Spine 1998 23 (18): 1937 – 1945

Radebold A, Cholewicki J, Panjabi MM, Patel TC. Muscle response pattern to sudden trunk loading in healthy individuals and in patients with chronic low back pain. Spine 2000 25 (8):947 – 954

Radebold A, Cholewicki J, Polzhofer GK, Greene HS. Impaired postural control of the lumbar spine is associated with delayed muscle response times in patients with chronic idiopathic low back pain. Spine 2001 26 (7):724 – 730

Ramsbacher J, Theallier-Janko A, Stoltenburg-Didinger G, Brock M. Ultrastructural changes in paravertebral muscles associated with degenerative spondylolisthesis. Spine 2001 26 (20):2180 – 2185

Rantanen J, Hurme M, Falck B, Alaranta H, Nykvist F, Lehto M, Einola S, Kalimo H. The lumbar multifidus muscle five years after surgery for a lumbar intervertebral disc herniation. Spine 1993 18 (5):568 – 574

Richardson C, Jull G, Hodges P, Hides J(a). Therapeutic exercise for spinal segmental stabilization in low back pain. 1999 Churchill Livingstone, Edinburgh

Richardson C, Jull G, Hodges P, Hides J(b). Therapeutic exercise for spinal segmental stabilization in low back pain. 1999 Churchill Livingstone, Edinburgh pp 129 – 138

Riihimaki H. Low-back pain, its origin and risk indicators. 1991 Scand J Work Environ Health 17 (2):81-90

Roland M, Fairbank, J. The Roland-Morris Disability Questionnaire and the Oswestry Disability Questionnaire. Spine 2000 25 (24):3115 - 3124

Salter RB. Textbook of disorders and injuries of the musculoskeletal system, 3rd Ed. 1999 Lippincott Williams & Wilkins, Philadelphia p. 275

Sapsford RR, Hodges PW, Richardson CA, Cooper DH, Markwell SJ, Jull GA. Co-activation of the abdominal and pelvic floor muscles during voluntary exercises. Neurourol Urodyn. 2001 20 (1):31-42

Schultz A, Warwick D, Berkson M, Nachemson A. Mechanical property of the human lumbar spine motion segments; Part 1. Responses in flexion, extension, lateral

188

bending and torsion. J Biomed Engineering 1979 (101):46 - 52

Schultz IZ, Crook JM, Berkowitz J, Meloche GR, Milner R, Zuberier OA, Meloche W. Biopsychosocial multivariate predictive model of occupational low back disability. Spine 2002 27 (23):2720 – 2725

Shaughnessy M, Caulfield B. A pilot study to investigate the effect of lumbar stabilisation exercise training on functional ability and quality of life in patient's with chronic low back pain. Int J Rehab Res 2004 27 (4): 297 - 301

Sihvonen T, Herno A, Paljarvi L, Airaksinen O, Partanen J, Tapaninaho A. Local denervation atrophy of paraspinal muscles in postoperative failed back syndrome. Spine 1993 18 (5):575 – 581

Silfies SP, Squillante D, Maurer P, Wescott S, Karduna AR. Trunk muscle recruitment in specific chronic low back pain populations. Clin Biomech *in press*

Sirca A, Kostevc V. The fibre type composition of thoracic and lumbar paravertebral muscles in man. J Anat 1985 141:131 - 137

Smith BH, Elliot AM, Hannaford PC, Chambers WA, Smith WC. Factors related to the onset and persistence of chronic back pain in the community. Spine 2004 29 (9): 1032 – 1040

Solomonow M, Zhou BH, Harris M, Lu Y, Baratta RV. The ligamento-muscular stabilizing system of the spine. Spine 1998 23 (23):2552 – 2562

Solomonow M, Zhou BH, Baratta RV, Lu Y, Harris M. Biomechanics of increased exposure to lumbar injury caused by cyclic loading: Part I. Loss of reflexive muscular stabilization. Spine 1999 24 (23):2426 – 2434

Spencer JD, Hayes KC, Alexander IJ. Knee joint effusion and quadriceps reflex inhibition in man. Arch Phys Med Rehabil. 1984 65(4):171-177

Spengler DM, Bigos SJ, Martin NA, Zeh J, Fisher L, Nachemson A. Back injuries in industry: a retrospective study. I. Overview and cost analysis. Spine 1986 11(3):241-245

Spitzer WO, LeBlanc FE, Dupuis M, et al. Scientific approach to the assessment and management of activity-related spinal disorders: A monograph for clinicians. Report of the Quebec Task Force on Spinal Disorders. Spine 1987 12 (Suppl):S1 – 59

Stokes IAF, Gardner-Morse M. Spinal stiffness increases with axial load: another stabilizing consequence of muscle action. J EMG Kines 2003 (13):397 – 402

Stokes IA, Henry SM, Single RM. Surface EMG electrodes do not accurately record from lumbar multifidus muscles. Clin Biomech 2003 18 (1):9 - 13

Taylor H, McGregor AH, Medhi-Zadeh S, Richards S, Kahn N, Zadeh JA, Hughes SPF. The impact of self-retaining retractors on the paraspinal muscles during posterior spinall surgery. Spine 2002 27 (24):2758 – 2762

Terry W, Higgs J. Educational programmes to develop clinical reasoning skills. Australian Phys J 1993 39 (1):47– 51

van den Hoogen HJM, Koes BW, Deville W, van Eijk JTM, Bouter LM. The prognosis of low back pain in general practice. Spine 1997 22 (13):1515 – 1521

van Dieen JH(a), Cholewicki J, Radebold A. Trunk muscle recruitment patterns in patients with low back pain enhance the stability of the lumbar spine. Spine 2003 28 (8): 834 – 841

van Dieen JH(b), Selen LPJ, Colewicki J. Trunk muscle activation in low back pain patients, an analysis of the literature. J EMG Kines 2003 (13): 333 – 351

van Tulder, M. Chronic back pain: Presentation of the new European guidelines. *In*, Proceedings of the 5th Interdisciplinary Congress on Low Back & Pelvic Pain. Melbourne, 2004

Varamini A, Jam B (a). A need for a shared paradigm in the physical therapy classification and treatment of mechanical low back pain: Part 1: Limitations of the patho-anatomical approach. Ortho Div Rev 2005 Mar/April: 40 - 43

Varamini A, Jam B (b). A need for a shared paradigm in the physical therapy classification and treatment of mechanical low back pain: Part 2: Practice guideline versus classification systems. Ortho Div Rev 2005 Mar/April: 44 - 51

Videman T, Battie MC, Gibbons LE, Maravilla K, Manninen H, Kaprio J. Associations between back pain history and lumbar MRI findings. Spine 2003 28 (6):582 – 588

Vleeming A, Snijders CJ, Stoeckart R, Mens JMA. A new light on low back pain. The self-locking mechanism of the sacroiliac joints and its implications for sitting, standing and walking. *In*, Proceedings of the 2nd Interdisciplinary World Congress on Low Back Pain. 1995 pp. 149 – 168

Von Korff M, Saunders K. The course of back pain in primary care. Spine 1996 21 (24):2833 – 2837

Waddell G. A new clinical model for the treatment of low-back pain. Spine 1987 12 (7):632 - 644

White AA, Panjabi MM. Clinical biomechanics of the spine. 1978 Lippincott, Philadelphia; p. 194

Wilke HJ, Wolf S, Claes LE, Arand M, Wiesend A. Stability increase of the lumbar spine with different muscle groups. Spine 1995 20 (2):192 – 198

Wilke HJ, Rohlmann A, Neller S, Graichen F, Claes L, Bergmann G. A novel approach to determine trunk muscle forces during flexion and extension. A comparison of data from an *in vitro* experiment and *in vivo* measurements. Spine 2003 28 (23):2585 – 2593

Wolf SL, Wolf LB, Segal RL. The relationship of extraneous movements to lumbar paraspinal muscle activity: Implications for EMG biofeedback training applications to low back pain patients. Biofeedback & Self-Regulation 1989 14 (1):63 - 74

Wright, A. Hypoalgesia post-manipulative therapy: a review of a potential neurophysiological mechanism. Man Ther 2000 1(1):11 - 16

Yoshihara K, Shirai Y, Kakayama Y, Uesaka S. Histochemical changes in the multifidus muscle in patients with lumbar intervertebral disc herniation. Spine 2001 26 (6):622 – 626

Zhao WP, Kawaguchi Y, Matsui H, Kanamori M, Kimura T. Histochemistry and morphology of the multifidus muscle in lumbar disc herniation. Comparative study between diseased and normal sides. Spine 2000 25 (17):2191 – 2199

index

Z

about the authors

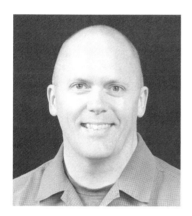

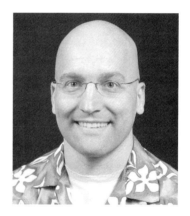

Rick graduated from the University of Toronto's Department of Physical Therapy in 1994. His clinical and research interests include the anatomical and motor control-related aspects of lumbar and shoulder pathology. He has taught continuing education courses for physiotherapists across Canada and in the United States since 1997. Rick has authored both peer-reviewed research as well as books on the topics of low back pain and 'core' conditioning for competitive athletes. *Physiotherapeutic Management of Lumbar Spine Pathology* is his third book.

David graduated from the Dalhousie University School of Physiotherapy in 1994, then pursued a manual therapy education, passing his Canadian Physiotherapy Asssociation ortho-paedic manipulation exams in 2002. He has since gone on to graduate studies with Dr. Paul Hodges in Brisbane, Australia. His research has been presented at major scientific conferences and published in peer-reviewed journals. David teaches continuing education courses for physiotherapists through the Atlantic Manual Therapy Institute.

novont health publishing

Current Titles:

Spinal Stabilization - The New Science of Back Pain, 2nd Edition

Author, Rick Jemmett
ISBN 09688715-1-8
Release Date   April 15, 2003

Spinal Stabilization Poster Set

Release Date   June 1, 2003

A Primer on Musculoskeletal Examination

Author, Evelyn Sutton, MD, FRCPC
ISBN 0-9688715-4-2
Release Date   June 15, 2004

The Athlete's Ball

Author, Rick Jemmett
ISBN 0-9688715-5-0
Release Date   August 1, 2004

Physiotherapeutic Management of Lumbar Spine Pathology: An evidence-based, best practice clinical model

Authors, David MacDonald & Rick Jemmett
ISBN 09688715-2-6
Release Date   June 1, 2005

For purchase enquiries regarding these publications, please contact:

novont health publishing limited

5595 Fenwick Street
PO Box 27069
Halifax, NS CAN   B3H 4M8
Telephone 902.423.4344   Facsimile 902.423.3477

For further information, please visit our website
novonthealth.com

Distributed by:

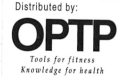

Tools for fitness
Knowledge for health

PO Box 47009
Minneapolis, Minnesota
55447-0009   USA

800-367-7393
(763) 553-0452